ALSO BY SANDEEP JAUHAR

Doctored

Intern

HEART

HEART

A History

SANDEEP JAUHAR

Farrar, Straus and Giroux   New York

Farrar, Straus and Giroux
175 Varick Street, New York 10014

Portions of this book originally appeared in different form
in *The New York Times* and *The New England Journal of Medicine*.

Library of Congress Cataloging-in-Publication Data
Names: Jauhar, Sandeep, 1968– author.
Title: Heart : a history / Sandeep Jauhar.
Description: First edition. | New York : Farrar, Straus and Giroux, 2018. |
    Includes index.
Identifiers: LCCN 2017055262 | ISBN 9780374168650 (hardcover)
Subjects: | MESH : Heart | Heart Diseases | Cardiologists | Cardiology |
    Personal Narratives
Classification: LCC QP111.4 | NLM WG 200 | DDC 612.1/7—dc23
LC record available at https://lccn.loc.gov/2017055262

Designed by Jonathan D. Lippincott

Our books may be purchased in bulk for promotional, educational, or business
use. Please contact your local bookseller or the Macmillan Corporate and
Premium Sales Department at 1-800-221-7945, extension 5442,
or by e-mail at MacmillanSpecialMarkets@macmillan.com.

www.fsgbooks.com
www.twitter.com/fsgbooks • www.facebook.com/fsgbooks

3   5   7   9   10   8   6   4   2

The names and identifying characteristics of some persons described
in this book have been changed.

For Pia, my heart

The animating spark of the body, nurse of its life, the creative principle and harmonizing bond of the senses; the central link in the human structure . . . mainstay of our nature, king, governor, creator.

    —Bernard Silvester, twelfth-century poet and philosopher

Contents

HEART

Prologue: CT Scan

I'd been getting short of breath. When I walked up the scuffed steps to my fourth-floor office, I had to stop to rest. Sometimes, at night, I would start to wheeze as my airways congested with mucus, and I'd break into fits of cough. As a physician, I was privileged to have been a first responder on 9/11, but many of us who had been at Ground Zero were reporting respiratory problems. So I went to my friend Seth, a pulmonologist, for an evaluation. He ordered pulmonary function tests, in which I sat in a glass-walled booth and blew hard into a plastic tube. Airflow and lung volumes were normal. Seth diagnosed me with acid reflux, a common cause of chronic cough, and prescribed a daily antacid. But I persuaded him to order a CT scan of my chest. My symptoms seemed out of proportion to his benign diagnosis. I was worried that my lungs had been damaged by the smoke and dust I'd inhaled downtown.

As Seth predicted, the CT scan revealed normal lungs. However, an incidental finding caught my eye. "Coronary artery calcifications are noted," the report offhandedly stated. Coronary calcium is a marker of atherosclerosis, hardening of the arteries. It had been reported as an incidental finding on countless CT scans of my older patients over the years, and I'd scarcely paid any attention. But now, at age forty-five, I wanted to know more. How much calcium was present, and where, exactly? A radiologist informed me that the scan I'd had did not have the resolution to answer these questions.

On my computer, I pulled up a Framingham calculator, a tool designed to estimate one's risk of a heart attack within the next ten years. I put in my height and weight, blood pressure and cholesterol, and the fact that I am a nonsmoker and don't have diabetes. The program spit out a ten-year risk of a heart attack of 2 percent and of any cardiovascular event (including angina and stroke) of about 7 percent. Reassuringly low. However, I also knew that for an Indian immigrant with a strong family history of heart disease, the calculation probably underestimated the true risk.

My brother, Rajiv, also a cardiologist, suggested a treadmill stress test, but I was playing tennis on weekends without any symptoms. A stress test would only detect coronary blockages greater than 70 percent, and I was pretty sure my disease was not that advanced. So I opted for a special, noninvasive CT angiogram to look into my coronaries. Every Father's Day I received spam e-mail about this test. "Make sure Dad is not among the hundreds of thousands of men in America who appear healthy but are actually a ticking time bomb." Strange to think that I might now be one of those men. I called Dr. Trost, the cardiac radiologist in our department, and scheduled the scan. She reassured me that I was at low risk for heart disease. "But for your peace of mind, you should probably have it," she said.

So, early one morning in June, I went for the test. While I lay on the gantry outside the C-shaped scanner, a tech inserted an IV in the back of my hand. The scan would have to resolve millimeter-sized plaque in a grapefruit-sized organ moving at a velocity of 200 millimeters per second. I was given an intravenous beta-blocker to slow down my heart to reduce image blur. A nitroglycerin tablet was also placed under my tongue to dilate my chest arteries so the scan could visualize them better. After a couple of preliminary images, a nurse injected X-ray-opaque dye into my vein. "You're going to feel warm all over," she said as I blushed, thinking I had wet myself. The final run-through took less than a minute.

After Dr. Trost reviewed the images, she called me into the reading room. The gray-and-white pictures were up on a large monitor. White specks, radiographic grit, were in all three of my coronary vessels. The main artery feeding my heart had a 30 to 50 percent obstruction near the opening and a 50 percent blockage in the midportion. There was minor plaque in the other two arteries, too. Sitting numbly in that dark room, I felt as if I were getting a glimpse of how I was probably going to die.

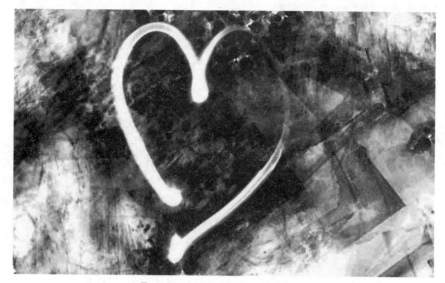

Fear Heart (Courtesy of Darian Barr)

Introduction:
The Engine of Life

There is nothing shameful about a heart attack.
—Susan Sontag, *Illness as Metaphor* (1978)

Perhaps the most consequential event in my life occurred fifteen years before I was born. On a sweltering July day in India in 1953, my paternal grandfather died suddenly. He was only fifty-seven. The circumstances were unusual, and like most family tragedies, ours has acquired a touch of myth. Everyone agrees that in the morning on the day he died, my grandfather was bitten by a snake coiled between sacks of grain in his little shop in Kanpur. He did not see the type of serpent, but snakebite is common in India, and by all accounts my grandfather was feeling fine when he came home for lunch. My father, who was almost fourteen, was going for an interview at Kanpur Agricultural College the following day, and my grandfather had planned to accompany him. They were sitting on the stone floor, inspecting my father's high school diploma, delighting in all the academic honors he'd received, when, midway through the meal, neighbors brought in the corpse of the shiny black cobra they claimed had bitten my grandfather. (It had been killed by a snake charmer summoned to the shop.) My grandfather took one look at it and went pale. "How can I survive this?" he said, before slumping to the floor. The neighbors exhorted him to say "Ram, Ram," a Hindu prayer, but his last words, lying on the floor, his eyes turning to glass, were "I wanted to take Prem to college."

A government ambulance used to make rounds in the village regularly. Around 7:00 p.m., several hours after my grandfather's collapse, it was flagged down on a routine drive. By then, rigor mortis had set in, traveling like a slow wave from my grandfather's neck and jaw into his limbs. The paramedics immediately declared my grandfather had passed—he had no heartbeat—but the family, in denial, insisted they take him (and the snake) to a British-built hospital about five miles away. A doctor there pronounced my grandfather dead on arrival.

"It was a heart attack," the doctor said, dispelling the family's belief that a snake had killed their elder. My grandfather had succumbed to the most common cause of death throughout the world, sudden cardiac death after a myocardial infarction, or heart attack, perhaps triggered in his case by fright over the snakebite. With nothing to be done, and the summer heat threatening to spoil the body, my grandfather was brought back to the village and cremated the following day. Before a garlanded casket set on a pyre soaked in oil, people beat their heads in grief under a light blue sky.

Listening to family lore, I grew up with a fear of the heart as the executioner of men in the prime of their lives. Because of the heart, you could be healthy and still die; it seemed like such a cheat. The apprehension was fed by our grandmother, who came to live with us in California in the early 1980s (until she got homesick and returned to the tiny village in Kanpur where her beloved husband had died). Even thirty years after his death, she still wrapped herself in white gossamer shawls that smelled of mothballs, befitting a widow. Once, at the Los Angeles Zoo, she bowed respectfully to the snake they brought around, clasping her hands and muttering a prayer before insisting we take her home. She was a strong-willed woman who ably took over the reins of the household after her husband died. And yet, like Miss Havisham, she spent her life in mourning over one freakish, incomprehensible incident. In India, snakes symbolize infinity and timelessness, as well as misfortune and death. To the end, in her mind, it was a venomous snake that killed her husband. And in a way, in the suddenness with which a heart attack can fell a healthy and vibrant life without warning, it was.

My maternal grandfather also fell victim to sudden cardiac death, though many years later. He was an army doctor who set up a successful private practice at his home in New Delhi. On a September morning in 1997, just after his eighty-third birthday, he woke up complaining of abdominal pain, which he attributed to an excess of food and scotch the night before. After a few minutes, he bellowed a loud groan and went unconscious; just like that, he was gone. He almost certainly had had a massive heart attack, but that wasn't what killed him. It was the ensuing arrhythmia—ventricular fibrillation, in which the heartbeat becomes chaotic—that prevented his heart from sustaining blood flow and life. When I talked to my mother about his death, she said she was sad that he died so suddenly. But she was thankful, too.

Thus, the human heart became an obsession for me, in no small part because of my family history. As a boy, I used to lie in bed and monitor the thudding in my own chest. I'd lie on my side, head in hand, and listen to the squirting pulse in my ears. I'd adjust the speed of the ceiling fan to synchronize with my heartbeat, in thrall to the two competing oscillators, so grateful that mine never took a rest.* I was fascinated by the heart's dichotomous nature: muscular, constantly toiling, and yet so vulnerable at the same time. Years later, when I became a heart-failure specialist, I reproduced this preoccupation in my

---

*Nineteenth-century scientists used a rotating wheel driven by a motor and synchronized to the cardiac cycle to detect small variations in the heart's rhythm.

children. When my son, Mohan, was small, we used to watch a PBS special on heart disease, in which a man having a heart attack develops cardiac arrest. In the back of an ambulance, he is shocked back to life with defibrillator paddles, his body violently jerking with the electrical discharge. Mohan would stare at the scene spellbound, often rewinding the tape, until I'd insist we turn it off, fearful of the impact on his developing mind. We'd watch it again the next day.

•

This book is about what the heart is, how it has been handled by medicine, and how we can most wisely live with—as well as by—our hearts in the future. The heart's vital importance to our self-understanding is no accident. If the heart is the last major organ to stop working, it is also the first to develop—starting to beat approximately three weeks into fetal life, even before there is blood to pump. From birth until death, it beats nearly three billion times. The amount of work it performs is mind-boggling. Each heartbeat generates enough force to circulate blood through approximately 100,000 miles of vessels. The amount of blood that passes through an average adult heart in a week could fill a backyard swimming pool. But the life that it sustains can quickly be taken away. When the heart stops, death is instantaneous. If life is a continuous struggle against the inexorable march of entropy, then the heartbeat is at the core of that conflict. By purveying energy to our cells, it counteracts our tendency toward dissipation and disarray.

More than anything, the heart wants to beat; this purpose is built into its very structure. Heart cells grown in a petri dish start to contract spontaneously, seeking out other cells (through electrical connections called gap junctions) to synchronize in their rhythmic dance. In this sense, cardiac cells—and the organ they create—are social entities. The heart can continue to beat for days, even weeks, after an animal has died. In a laboratory, the French Nobel laureate Alexis Carrel showed that properly nourished chick heart tissue cultured on a medium of blood plasma and water will pulsate for months and can remain alive for more than twenty years, much longer than the normal life span of its host. This is a unique property of the heart. The brain and other vital organs cannot function without a beating heart, but a beating heart does not depend on a functioning brain, at least not in the short term. Moreover, the heart doesn't just pump blood to other organs; it pumps blood to *itself.* We cannot see our own eyes. We must struggle to use our minds to change our way of thinking. But the heart is different. In a sense, and unlike any other organ, the heart is self-sustaining.

Of all the connections of the heart—to emotions, to thought—the link between the heartbeat and life is perhaps the strongest. We associate the heart with life because, like life itself, the heart is dynamic. From second to second, and on a macroscopic scale, the heart is the only organ that discernibly moves. Through its murmurings, it speaks to us; through its synchronized contractions, it broadcasts an electrical signal several thousand times more powerful than any other in the body. Over the centuries, disparate cultures have viewed the heart as the source of a life-giving force that was to be culled or harvested. In ancient Egypt, the heart was the only organ that was left in the body during mummification because it was believed to play a central role in the rebirth of an individual after death.* In a scene often depicted in Egyptian mythology, the heart of a deceased person is weighed on a scale balanced by a feather or statuette representing truth and divine law. If the heart balanced

---

*The kidneys were also left behind, probably because their location in the body made removal difficult. One can almost hear the words of the recently departed Egyptian, bowed in submission, written on the papyrus: "O my heart which I had upon earth, do not rise up against me as a witness . . . Do not speak against me concerning what I have done." Through the Middle Ages, the hearts of kings and princes were still often buried separately, and as recently as 1989 the queen of Hungary chose to have her heart interred in a monastery in Switzerland where her husband's heart also lay.

evenly, it was considered pure and returned to its owner. But if it proved laden with sin, it was devoured by a monstrous chimera, and the deceased was banished to the underworld. Three thousand years later, in elaborate hilltop ceremonies, the Aztecs opened the chests of slaves with flint knives and ripped out their still-beating hearts as offerings to their idols. In Western fairy tales, witches seeking immortality consumed the hearts of innocents. In *Snow White*, for example, the evil queen insists the hunter cut out the girl's heart to ensure that she is really dead. Even today, when brain death has become a widely accepted sign of demise, people continue to associate a heartbeat with viability. Families come up to me in the intensive care unit and say, "His heart is beating. How could he be dead?"

The sanguine dance must eventually come to an end. Cardiovascular disease claims 18 million lives—nearly one-third of all deaths—across the globe each year. Since 1910, heart disease has been the number one killer in the United States. Today 62 million Americans (and more than 400 million worldwide, including 7 million in the United Kingdom) suffer from heart disease.

The second most common cause of death in America is cancer, but heart disease and cancer could hardly be more different. In cancer, cells divide madly, migrate wildly, invade mercilessly, in a sort of hard-charging pollution of the body. Heart disease is different: cleaner, stricter, less ambiguous, more comprehensible. Cancer patients, Susan Sontag wrote, are stained and fragmented. Cardiac patients, she said, often stand tall, seemingly healthy, like my grandfather, until they die.

The numbers could be even worse. Cardiovascular deaths in America have actually declined by almost 60 percent since the mid-1960s. From 1970 to 2000, the average life span in the United States increased by six years. Two-thirds of this increase in longevity came from advances in cardiovascular treatments. (In recent years there has been decreasing life span in middle-aged whites for non-cardiovascular reasons.) Although more than 60 percent of Americans will develop some form of cardiovascular disease in their lifetime, less than a third will die of it, so we know our treatments are effective. The twentieth century will go down in history as one in which the great scourge of cardiovascular disease finally began to come under control.

There is a downside to this success, of course. Patients who once might have died of heart disease now must live with it, though often in an enervated state, a fraction of their former selves. Every year more than half a million Americans develop congestive heart failure, in which the heart weakens or stiffens to the point that it cannot properly pump blood to meet the energy demands of the body. Heart failure is now the number one reason patients over sixty-five years old are hospitalized, and most patients still die within five years of diagnosis. Ironically, as we become more adept at treating heart disease, the set of people who are ill with it is growing.

The cardiovascular situation in America is likely going to get worse in the coming years. Adherence to a heart-healthy lifestyle has decreased. In aggregate, Americans have become more obese and sedentary, and smoking rates have hardly changed in the past two decades. An autopsy study in the *Archives of Internal Medicine* suggests that 80 percent of Americans sixteen to sixty-four years old have at least the beginnings of coronary artery disease. These findings indicate that the four-decade-long decline in heart disease may be coming to a screeching halt. We will need new ways to cope with this threat.

In the pages that follow, I will examine the emotional and scientific dimensions of an organ that has intrigued and eluded philosophers and physicians for centuries. No other organ—perhaps no other object in human life —is so imbued with metaphor and meaning. The history I will describe is not one of uninterrupted progress, but it is one that, in fits and starts, has solved major challenges, helping countless people survive a disease that was once considered terminal. It is a grand story—

from the natural philosophers who dwelled on the heart's meta-phorical meanings, to William Harvey and the discovery of circulation, to large-scale endeavors like the Framingham Heart Study that explored the causes of heart disease, to modern surgical techniques and technologies that even a century ago, because of the heart's exalted status in human culture, were considered taboo.

The twelfth-century Christian mystic Hildegard of Bingen once wrote, "The soul sits at the center of the heart, as though in a house." In many ways, the heart does resemble a house. It is divided into multiple chambers, separated by doors. The walls have a characteristic texture. The house is old, designed over many millennia. Hidden from view are the wires and pipes that keep it functioning. And though the house has no intrinsic meaning, it carries meaning because of the meanings we attri-bute to it. The heart was once considered the center of human action and thought—the source of courage, desire, ambition, and love. Even if those connotations are outdated, they are still deeply relevant to how we think about this organ and how it shapes our lives.

PART I

Metaphor

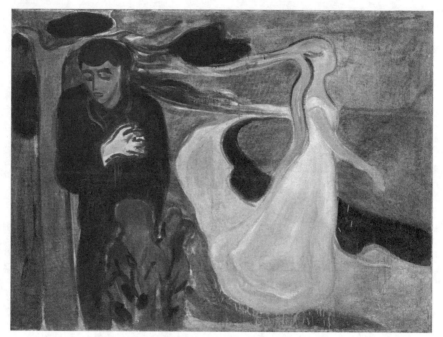

Separation, Edvard Munch, 1896, oil on canvas, 96.5 × 127 cm (Munch Museum, Oslo [MM M 00024]; photograph © Munch Museum)

1

A Small Heart

You can die of a broken heart—it's scientific fact—and my
heart has been breaking since that very first day we met. I
can feel it now, aching deep behind my rib cage the way
it does every time we're together, beating a desperate
rhythm: *Love me. Love me. Love me.*

—Abby McDonald, *Getting Over
Garrett Delaney* (2012)

When I was fifteen, I had to do a research project for my high
school biology class. I decided to measure the electrical signal
from the heart of a live frog. To do the experiment, I was going
to have to pith the animal—sever its spinal cord while it was still
alive, thus paralyzing it—before cutting it open. I borrowed an
oscilloscope to measure current, a voltage amplifier, and some
red and black electrodes. My science teacher, Mr. Crandall, said
it was an impressive project for a high school junior.

But first I had to collect some frogs. With a fishing net in
one hand and my bicycle handlebars in the other, I set off for
the woods near my house in Southern California. It was a late
Friday afternoon in early spring, and birds were singing petu-
lantly. The road was wet. My bicycle tires made gritty sounds
in the gravelly mud.

My destination was a small pond, no bigger than a back-yard swimming pool. The surface was blanketed with leaves, dragonflies, and interconnecting swaths of green muck. I plod-ded along the bank, my sneakers sinking ever so slightly into the mud. Then, through a parting in the algae, I beheld a wondrous world of darting tadpoles and surging tree frogs. I plunged my net, a white mesh at the end of a three-foot wooden pole, into the water and dragged it along the viscous bottom. When I pulled it out, a small yellow frog was caught in the net-ting. I dropped it (along with a few leaves) into a garbage bag. With a few more sweeps, I collected more frogs, about six in all. I poked tiny holes in the plastic bag with the tip of a pencil and tied off the top. Then, after stuffing the bag into my back-pack, I rode home.

I dropped the bike at the side of the house and unlatched the wooden door leading to the backyard. Weeds peeked out of cracks in the cement path. Beside the covered patio was a small lemon tree. The fact that it was there always made me feel as if my backyard were a better, freer place than it really was. By then, darkness was approaching, replacing the jaundiced sky. From the kitchen, my mother called out to me to come in for dinner. I left the bag with the frogs on the patio. Inside, my mother asked me if I was going to feed the animals. I told her there was no point because they were going to be sacrificed anyway.

Animal circulation, I'd learned from Mr. Crandall, evolved over millions of years. Mollusks and worms have a low-pressure, open circulation to ferry nutrients and waste. Larger animals developed tube-shaped vessels and pumps of growing com-plexity to circulate blood at higher pressure, thus enabling oxy-gen and nutrient delivery over longer distances. Fish hearts have two chambers; frog hearts have three. Human hearts are more intricate, with four chambers: two atria (the collecting compartments) and two ventricles (the pumps). Frogs require less oxygen than humans because they do not try to maintain a constant internal temperature. Unlike the humans who dis-sect them, frogs are cold-blooded.

The next day, a Saturday, I took the garbage bag, my electrical apparatus, a scalpel, and a dissection tray and sat down on a plastic stool under our rusting swing set. In 1856, 127 years earlier, the anatomists Rudolf von Kölliker and Heinrich Müller measured the electric current of a frog's heartbeat by passing the current down electrodes connected to a magnet, which produced a force that deflected a needle. With some modern technology, this was essentially the experiment I was going to try to replicate. I hooked up the electrodes to the voltage source to test the circuit, getting a clean 60-hertz signal on the oscilloscope. Because the electrode tips were fat and blunt, I wasn't sure they'd make proper contact if the frog's heart was too small, but that weekend was the best time for me to get the experiment done, so I decided to proceed anyway.

I retrieved a frog from the depths of the bag. Grasping it firmly with my hand, I gently applied the scalpel to the beige skin on its back. It kicked its legs wildly, struggling to get free. When I inadvertently relaxed my grip, it got away, hopping around in the dry grass until I scooped it up. Squeezing its hip and hind legs securely until it stopped resisting, I tried again. By this point my own heart was popping against my breastbone, trying to break free. I pushed the tip of the scalpel a few millimeters through the soft foramen magnum and into the base of the skull. The frog struggled, so I pushed harder, feeling the cartilaginous carapace reluctantly give way. I must have been holding my breath—or perhaps hyperventilating—because tiny grains of black began to mottle my vision. I rattled the tip violently back and forth, nearly decapitating the animal. When I placed it in the dissection tray, it tried to drag itself to the edge. It gave one more weak jump before it went limp.

I made a linear incision along the chest, which bled clear, viscous liquid. The heart was still beating, as far as I could tell—though it was hard to be sure, shrouded as it was by other thoracic structures. To clear the field, I tore out these organs with my fingers. By then my tears were flowing fast. The electrode tips were way too big, nearly the size of the heart itself. Nevertheless, in a panic, I directed them at the pea-sized organ, forgetting that they were still hooked up to the battery. When they made contact, an electrical spark crackled, singeing the chest. It smelled awful, even worse than the formaldehyde-soaked specimens in Mr. Crandall's storage locker. By the time my mother came outside, I was bawling. I had tortured the poor creature, and moreover had nothing to show for it. My mother surveyed the scene carefully. Then, with her usual scolding sympathy, she said, "You should do a different experiment, son. Your heart is too small for this."

The next day, I steeled myself to try again, but when I went to retrieve another frog, the bag was empty; the frogs had disappeared. I still don't know how they escaped (and neither did my mother). With no original data, I filled my paper with figures from textbooks. I got a B. Disappointed, I asked Mr. Crandall why. He said it was because I had learned nothing new.

•

If the heart bestows life and death, it also instigates metaphor: it is a vessel that fills with meaning. The fact that my mother associated my lack of courage with a small heart is no surprise; the heart has always been linked to bravery. During the Renaissance, the heart on a coat of arms was a symbol of faithfulness and courage. Even the word "courage" derives from the Latin *cor*, which means "heart." A person with a small heart is easily frightened. Discouragement or fear is expressed as a loss of heart.

This metaphor exists across cultures. After my grandfather died, my father, only fourteen, enrolled at Kanpur Agricultural College, the first in his family to pursue higher education. Every morning he would walk six kilometers to the academy because the family could not afford a bicycle. On the way home, lugging his bag of borrowed books, he would meet my grandmother at an appointed spot on the dusty road. When he would complain of feeling tired or overwhelmed, she would admonish her grieving boy to show strength. "*Dil himmauth kar*," she'd say. Take heart.

Shakespeare explored this motif in his tragedies. In *Antony and Cleopatra*, Dercetas describes the warrior Antony's suicide by the hand that "with the courage which the heart did lend it, splitted the heart." Antony was distraught over what he believed to be Cleopatra's treachery, and in describing Antony's heartbreak, Shakespeare refers to another conception of the heart: as the locus of romantic love. "I made these wars for Egypt and the Queen," Antony declares, "whose heart I thought I had, for she had mine." As the critic Joan Lord Hall writes, Antony is conflicted over two very different conceptions of the metaphorical heart. In the end, his craving for battlefield glory overwhelms his desire for passionate fulfillment and leads to his self-destruction.

The richness and breadth of human emotions are perhaps what distinguish us most from other animals, and throughout history and across many cultures, the heart has been thought of as the place where those emotions reside. The word "emotion" derives from the French verb *émouvoir*, meaning "to stir up," and perhaps it is only logical that emotions would be linked to an organ characterized by its agitated movement. The idea that the heart is the locus of emotions has a history spanning from the ancient world. But this symbolism has endured.

If we ask people which image they most associate with love, there is no doubt that the valentine heart would top the list. The ♥ shape, called a cardioid, is common in nature. It appears in the leaves, flowers, and seeds of many plants, including silphium, which was used for birth control in the early Middle Ages and may be the reason why the heart became associated with sex and romantic love (though the heart's resemblance to the vulva probably also has something to do with it). Whatever the reason, hearts began to appear in paintings of lovers in the thirteenth century. (These depictions at first were restricted to aristocrats and members of the court—hence the term "courtship.") Over time the pictures came to be colored red, the color of blood, a symbol of passion. Later, heart-shaped ivy, reputed for its longevity and grown on tombstones, became an emblem of eternal love. In the Roman Catholic Church, the ♥ shape became known as the Sacred Heart of Jesus; adorned with thorns and emitting ethereal light, it was an insignia of monastic love. Devotion to the Sacred Heart reached peak intensity in Europe in the Middle Ages. In the early fourteenth century, for instance, Heinrich Seuse, a Dominican monk, in a fit of pious fervor (and gruesome self-mutilation), took a stylus to his own chest to engrave the name of Jesus onto his heart. "Almighty God," Seuse wrote, "give me strength this day to carry out my desire, for thou must be chis-eled into the core of my heart." The bliss of having a visible pledge of oneness with his true love, he added, made the very pain seem like a "sweet delight." When his wounds healed in the spongy tissue, the sacred name was written in letters "the width of a cornstalk and the length of the joint of [a] little fin-ger." This association between the heart and different types of love has withstood modernity. When Barney Clark, a retired dentist with end-stage heart failure, received the first perma-nent artificial heart in Salt Lake City, Utah, on December 1, 1982, his wife of thirty-nine years asked the doctors, "Will he still be able to love me?"

Today we know that emotions do not reside in the heart per se, but we nevertheless continue to subscribe to the heart's sym-bolic connotations. Heart metaphors abound in everyday life and language. To "take heart" is to have courage. To "speak from the heart" conveys sincerity. We say we "learned by heart" what we have understood thoroughly or committed to mem-ory. To "take something to heart" reflects worry or sadness. If your "heart goes out to someone," you sympathize with his or her problems. Reconciliation or repentance requires a "change of heart."

Like the biological heart, the metaphorical heart has both

size and shape. A bighearted person is generous; a small-hearted person is selfish (though when my mother said I had a small heart, I believe she meant I had a surfeit of compassion). The metaphorical heart is also a material entity. It can be made of gold, stone, even liquid (for example, being poured when we confess something). The metaphorical heart also possesses temperature—warm, cold, hot—as well as a characteristic geography. The center of a place is its heart. Your "heart of heart," as Hamlet tells Horatio, is the place of your most sacred feelings. To "get to the heart" of something is to find out what is truly important, and just as the statue or monument at the heart of a city often has something to do with love, bravery, or courage, so too it is with the human heart.

●

Over the years, I have learned that the proper care of my patients depends on trying to understand (or at least recognize) their emotional states, stresses, worries, and fears. There is no other way to practice heart medicine. For even if the heart is not the seat of the emotions, it is highly responsive to them. In this sense, a record of our emotional life *is* written on our hearts. Fear and grief, for example, can cause profound myocardial injury. The nerves that control unconscious processes, such as the heartbeat, can sense distress and trigger a maladaptive fight-or-flight response that signals blood vessels to constrict, the heart to gallop, and blood pressure to rise, resulting in damage.

In other words, it is increasingly clear that the biological heart is extraordinarily sensitive to our emotional system—to the metaphorical heart, if you will.

In the early part of the twentieth century, Karl Pearson, a biostatistician studying cemetery headstones, noticed that husbands and wives tend to die within a year of each other. This finding supports what we now know to be true: heartbreak can cause heart attacks; loveless marriages can lead to chronic and acute heart disease. A 2004 study of nearly thirty thousand

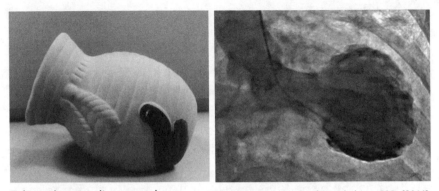

Takotsubo cardiomyopathy (from *International Journal of Cardiology* 209 [2016]: 196–205)

patients in fifty-two countries found that psychosocial factors, including depression and stress, were as strong risk factors for heart attacks as high blood pressure and nearly as important as diabetes. The heart might be a pump, but it is certainly not a simple one, and it is most definitely an emotional one.

There is a heart disorder first recognized about two decades ago called takotsubo cardiomyopathy, or the broken-heart syndrome, in which the heart acutely weakens in response to extreme stress or grief, such as after a romantic breakup or the death of a spouse. Patients (almost always women, for unclear reasons) develop symptoms that mimic those of a heart attack. They may develop chest pain and shortness of breath, even heart failure. On an echocardiogram, the heart muscle appears stunned, frequently ballooning into the shape of a *takotsubo*, a Japanese octopus-trapping pot with a wide bottom and a narrow neck.

Though we don't know exactly why this happens, the abnormal shape seems to reflect the distribution of adrenaline receptors in the normal heart. High adrenaline damages heart cells. Areas with higher receptor density (such as the apex, or bottom, of the heart) are more affected and therefore suffer the most damage. Though takotsubo cardiomyopathy often resolves within a few weeks, in the acute period it can cause heart failure, life-threatening arrhythmias, even death. The first studies of this disorder were in the early 1980s on victims of emotional or physical trauma (robbery, attempted murder) who seemed to die not from their injuries but from cardiac causes. Autopsies showed telltale signs of heart injury and cell death.

Takotsubo cardiomyopathy is the archetype of a disease that is controlled by interactions between the emotions and the physical body. In no other condition do the biological and metaphorical hearts intersect so closely. The disorder can even occur when patients are not conscious of their grief. The husband of an elderly patient of mine had died. She was sad, of course, but accepting, maybe even a bit relieved: it had been a long illness; he had had dementia. But a week after the funeral, she looked at his picture and became tearful, and then she got chest pain, and with it came shortness of breath, distended neck veins, sweaty brow, a noticeable panting while she was quietly sitting in a chair: signs of congestive heart failure. On an ultrasound, her heart had weakened to less than half its normal function. But nothing on other tests was amiss—no sign of clogged arteries anywhere. Two weeks later, her emotional state had returned to normal and so, an ultrasound confirmed, had her heart.

Takotsubo cardiomyopathy has been reported in many stressful situations, including public speaking, gambling losses, domestic disputes, even a surprise birthday party. "Outbreaks" of it have even been associated with widespread social upheaval, such as after a natural disaster. For example, on October 23, 2004, a major earthquake registering 6.8 on the Richter scale devastated Niigata Prefecture on Honshu, the largest island in Japan. Thirty-nine people were killed, and more than three thousand were injured. Landslides forced the closure of two national highways, disrupting telephone service and power and water supplies. On the heels of this catastrophe, researchers found that there was a twenty-four-fold increase in the number of takotsubo cardiomyopathy cases in the Niigata district one

month after the earthquake, compared with a similar period
the year before. The residences of those affected were closely
correlated with the intensity of the tremor. In almost every
case, patients lived near the epicenter.

Using a nationwide database, scientists at the University of
Arkansas identified almost 22,000 patients diagnosed with
takotsubo cardiomyopathy in the United States in 2011. The
highest rate of cases, nearly triple the national average, was in
Vermont, where a tropical storm wreaked more damage that
year than in nearly a century. The second-highest rate was in
Missouri, where a massive tornado ripped through the town of
Joplin, killing at least 158 people. Though these geographic
areas were not the only ones hit by natural disasters that year,
the scientists noted that their populations were perhaps less prepared because of a lack of experience with disasters and thus
more vulnerable to the ensuing distress.

By now, these findings should not surprise. Heart problems, including sudden cardiac death, have long been reported
in individuals experiencing intense emotional disturbance—
turmoil in their metaphorical hearts. The most unusual disturbances may have especially dramatic effects. In his book *The
Lost Art of Healing*, the cardiologist Bernard Lown describes a
case from an Indian medical journal in which a prisoner is con-
demned to death by hanging. A physician persuades the prisoner to allow authorities to bleed him rather than hang him
because death by exsanguination is relatively painless. The
man is strapped to a cot and blindfolded. Then his arms and legs
are scratched, leading him to believe that he is bleeding. Lown
writes:

> Vessels filled with water were hung at each of the four
> bedposts and set up to drip in a basin on the floor. The
> water began to drip into the containers, initially fast,
> then progressively slowing [mimicking bleeding]. By de-
> grees the prisoner grew weaker, a condition reinforced

by the physician's intoning in a lower and lower voice. Finally the silence was absolute as the dripping of water ceased. Although the prisoner was a healthy young man, at the completion of the experiment, when the water flow stopped, he appeared to have fainted. On examination, however, he was found to be dead, despite not having lost a single drop of blood.

These types of "emotional" deaths have been observed for at least a century. In 1942, the Harvard physiologist Walter B. Cannon published a paper called "'Voodoo' Death" in which he described cases of death from fright in primitive people who believed they had been cursed, such as by a bone-pointing witch doctor or as a consequence of eating "taboo" fruit. In his book *The Australian Aboriginal*, published in 1925, the anthropologist Herbert Basedow wrote:

> The man who discovers that he is being boned by an enemy is, indeed, a pitiable sight. He stands aghast with his eyes staring at the treacherous pointer, and with his hands lifted to ward off the lethal medium, which he imagines is pouring into his body. His cheeks blanch, and his eyes become glassy, and the expression of his face becomes horribly distorted. He attempts to shriek but usually the sound chokes in his throat, and all that one might see is froth at his mouth. His body begins to tremble and his muscles twitch involuntarily. He sways backward and falls to the ground, and after a short time appears to be in a swoon. He finally composes himself, goes to his hut and there frets to death.

What these deaths had in common was the victims' absolute belief that there was an external force that could cause their demise and against which they were powerless to fight. This perceived lack of control, Cannon postulated, resulted in an unmitigated physiological response in which blood vessels constricted to such a degree that blood volume acutely dropped, blood pressure plummeted, the heart acutely weakened, and massive organ damage resulted from a lack of transported oxygen. Cannon believed that voodoo deaths were limited to primitive people "so superstitious, so ignorant, that they feel themselves bewildered strangers in a hostile world." But over the years these types of sudden deaths have been shown to affect all manner of modern people, too. A host of sudden-death syndromes have been identified today, including sudden death in middle-aged men (usually after myocardial infarction), sudden infant death syndrome, sudden unexpected nocturnal death syndrome, sudden death during natural catastrophe, sudden death associated with recreational drug abuse, sudden death in wild and domestic animals, sudden death during alcohol withdrawal, sudden death after a major loss, sudden death during panic attacks, and sudden death during war. Almost all occur because of a sudden stoppage of the heart.

This is what happened to my grandfather. His sudden death was likely caused by the intense fright he experienced when he saw the snake that bit him. But stress can have both acute and chronic effects, and so I believe the emotional conditions for his cardiac death were laid much earlier, during the tumultuous partition of India in the summer of 1947. My grandfather lived in a district in the Punjab province of what is today Pakistan, where he owned a land management business, hiring laborers to tend to large estates. With the end of British rule in August 1947, the long-standing animosity between Hindus and Muslims in Punjab, as in the rest of the Indian subcontinent, exploded. That year, six years before my grandfather died, the country was partitioned into India and West and East Pakistan (now called Bangladesh), along largely sectarian lines. The result was the largest mass migration in recorded history. Millions of Hindus trekked into India (my grandfather's family among them). Millions of Muslims went in the opposite direction. The violence on both sides was unimaginable, with massacres, rapes, abductions, and forced religious conversions. One victim was my grandfather's family's priest, whose throat was cut by a Muslim gang when he refused to say *"Allahu akbar."* "We had Oms," my father explains, pointing to a gray tattoo on his hand. "No question they would have killed us, too."

My grandfather and his family escaped to the border in bullock-driven carts along rutted roads, taking whatever they could bear. There was terrible bloodshed along the way. Villages were in flames; families left behind small children because they could not carry them. The Indian government had issued special armed escorts for teenage girls. Even so, some killed their own daughters to keep them from being raped.

That year, as the country was torn apart, more than one million people died, and fifty million Hindus, Muslims, and Sikhs were uprooted. The epicenter of the violence was in Punjab, but the shock waves resounded across the subcontinent. My grandfather and his family survived, but months of squalor in border camps, where cholera and dysentery were rampant, would claim the lives of my grandfather's mother and his one-year-old son.

The struggle and upheaval during the summer and fall of 1947 no doubt contributed to my grandfather's premature demise six years later. Reeling from the loss of his business, the family eventually settled into a one-bedroom flat in rural Kanpur. They had no furniture, electricity, or running water. My father did his homework under streetlamps; my grandmother prepared meals on a wood-and-dung-burning stove. My grandfather eventually scraped together enough money to open a small convenience shop that sold rice and other foodstuffs, where he worked virtually every waking hour. He was at that shop on the day he died.

•

The heart's physiological responses to emotions such as fright, fear, or joy are controlled by the autonomic nervous system, which regulates unconscious movements such as heartbeat and breathing. The autonomic nervous system has two divisions: the "sympathetic" system, which mediates the fight-or-flight reaction, using adrenaline to speed up the heart and increase blood pressure; and the "parasympathetic" system, which has the opposite effect, slowing respirations and heartbeat, lowering blood pressure, and promoting digestion. Both sympathetic and parasympathetic nerves travel along blood vessels and terminate in nerve cells within the heart to help regulate the heart's emotional reactions.

However, there is still a lot we do not understand about the effects of the autonomic nervous system on the heart. For instance, in 1957, Curt Richter, a scientist at Johns Hopkins, described experiments on wild rats in which the animals were dunked in a glass jar filled with water and sprayed by a narrow jet that precluded the animals from floating—in essence, waterboarding them. Wild rats are fierce, suspicious animals that react very negatively to any form of restraint. Not surprisingly, most rats rapidly drowned within minutes (though a few amazingly were able to swim for eighty or more hours before drowning).

When Richter measured the heartbeat of the drowning rats by means of electrodes inserted under the skin, he discovered to his surprise that the rate was not rapid, as would be expected from sympathetic overactivity. "Contrary to our expectations, the EKG records indicated that the rats succumbing promptly died with a *slowing* of the heart rate rather than with an acceleration," Richter wrote, suggesting parasympathetic activation. Moreover, drugs that increased parasympathetic activity accelerated these deaths; drugs that blocked this activity prevented them. Therefore, Richter concluded that the rats died as the result of parasympathetic, not sympathetic, overactivation. "The situation of these rats scarcely seems one demanding fight or flight—it is rather one of hopelessness; whether they are restrained in the hand or confined in the swimming jar, the rats are in a situation against which they have no defense." Richter further noted that teaching the rats that their situation was not hopeless—by releasing them from the jar at certain intervals, for example—caused them to become aggressive again and try to escape. He conjectured that hopelessness, leading to parasympathetic overactivity, was the reason that aborigines succumbed to voodoo death.

It is now believed that the seemingly contradictory conclusions of Cannon and Richter are both true and that life-threatening stress unleashes an autonomic storm on the heart that has both sympathetic and parasympathetic components. Both mechanisms have now been implicated in takotsubo cardiomyopathy. Which one predominates depends largely on the time elapsed after the stress. Early on, sympathetic effects are most important (cardiac arrhythmias, elevated blood pressure), while parasympathetic effects (slowing of the heartbeat, lowering of blood pressure) come to the fore later.

Interestingly, takotsubo cardiomyopathy can develop after a happy event, too, but the heart appears to react differently—ballooning in the midportion, for instance, rather than at the apex. Why different emotional precipitants result in different cardiac changes is a mystery. But today—perhaps as an ode to our ancient philosophers—we can acknowledge that even if our emotions are not located inside our hearts, the biological heart overlaps with its metaphorical counterpart in surprising and mysterious ways.

2

Prime Mover

The six planets orbit the sun, as though around their
heart, and give power to the sun and draw power from it:
as life winds around the heart and penetrates into it.
—Jakob Böhme, German theologian, *The Threefold
Life of Man* (1620)

My first few days in St. Louis were horribly muggy. Clothes
clung to my skin like plastic wrap, and the air was like a thick
meringue. So, the anatomy lab at the medical school was a
welcome sanctuary: cold and dry, with limestone floors and
twelve-foot ceilings and a giant multi-faucet sink in the middle
of the room, where we assembled in green scrubs three morn-
ings a week, like animals at a watering hole, to wash our hands.
Hanging in a corner was a plastic skeleton, like a prop in a campy
horror film. With the chill in the sterile chamber, I half expected
its teeth to start chattering.

It would be two years before we entered the hospital to do
clinical rotations. Until then, we would have to satisfy ourselves
with a human dissection. Our cadavers would soon be in sun-
dry states of dismemberment, their vital organs soaking in buck-
ets of formalin on the floor. But for those first few days after
school opened in August, they lay there untouched.

Mine rested on a steel gurney with rusted wheels, swathed in a white plastic bag containing a shallow puddle of reddish liquid. Sunken chest, light brown skin, distended belly: he was naked save for the tiny socks covering his feet like a baby's bootees and the cloth mask over his face, which would slip off every now and then, revealing a morbidly serene visage. He was probably in his mid-eighties, faintly hominid in appearance, with a balding scalp, a Punjabi beak nose, and wrinkled leathery cheeks. His tongue partially hung out of his mouth, conferring a look of mild bemusement. Yellowish plaque, matching his pallid skin, caked his front teeth. Moldy-looking scabs pocked his eyelids. His contracted body raised unnatural bumps under the plastic.

"Autopsy" means "to see for oneself," and that was exactly what we were supposed to do. But before we got started—before we even applied scalpel to skin—our ponytailed anatomy professor had us do an exercise. What could we surmise about our cadavers, he asked, with an external inspection? What clues were available about how they might have lived or died? The most obvious thing about mine was that he died old. Surgical scars—most prominently a long track down the middle of his breastbone, a remnant of open-heart surgery—indicated that he'd had access to health care. His clean nail beds meant he had been well-off, at least well enough to take care of himself (or to pay others to take care of him). Callused hands generally suggest blue-collar work. My cadaver's hands were smooth and polished. The feeding tube in his stomach implied his final days had been difficult, perhaps spent in a nursing home or some other full-time care facility. The edema in his limbs pointed to congestive heart failure. And the bulge in his abdomen? Probably a pacemaker.

It was a fascinating exercise, a reminder to us aspiring doctors that even as we tried to figure out how our cadavers had died, we should not forget to think about how they might have lived. Reflect on their lives, our professor intoned, even as you cut. I took note to do that.

Even from our first encounter, my cadaver confounded me. He was South Asian. In the culture I grew up in, people rarely donate their bodies to science; they belong to their loved ones. In his final decision—just before death—my cadaver likely defied the wishes of his family, his children, maybe even his wife. Why? I wondered. Of course, I would never know, but nonetheless I felt a sort of kinship to the body before me. The cadavers, our professor said, might remind us of a person we once knew—a close friend or relative who had passed away. Or perhaps a grandfather who lived only in stale stories.

That semester, I felt closer to my paternal grandfather than ever. It was hard not to make a comparison between him and my cadaver. Both were Indian, probably born around the same time, and probably victims of the same disease. But there was at least one major difference. One man lived a full life, at least beyond what could reasonably be expected. The other died suddenly, leaving behind a distraught family without mooring. One life was terminated prematurely. My grandfather never got the chance to see my father off to college or watch him develop into a successful plant geneticist. The other lingered on into old age—in part because of where my cadaver had lived, because he had benefited from extraordinary scientific advances, many of them spearheaded in America. In a way, his life wasn't over; he continued to leave a legacy as a physical textbook for the next generation of doctors. The most interesting thing about my nameless cadaver, I realized, was not why he had died but rather how he had managed to live for as long as he did, when for others the journey had ended so abruptly.

I'm embarrassed to admit it, but for those first few weeks I mostly watched as others dissected. Cadavers made me queasy, and my chatty fellow students' poring over the body, like forensic pathologists, did nothing to lessen the discomfort with dissection that I'd carried ever since my frog experiment. So I stood at the periphery, peeking over green-scrubbed shoulders at the Indian man glistening under the ceiling lights. Multicolored pins were soon sticking into his various bodily structures.

I imagined his last, bitter days in the hospital: swollen legs, boggy lungs, staring out the window as the death rattle of congestive heart failure began to set in. I pictured him, lips pursed, trying to resist as a nurse force-fed him medicated chocolate pudding, a documentary about the British East India Company playing muffled in the background. He must have scowled as the bittersweet dessert entered his mouth, resentful of the judgments the nurses were making of him, a shell of the man he once was. "I hope your father suffers like you are making me suffer," I could hear him say.

When we finally got to the dissection of the heart, I steeled myself and stepped up. It was the experience for which I had been waiting—for the better part of my life. The anatomy manual was terse: "Secure a handsaw and open the chest wall." The skin overlying my cadaver's ribs was like wet leather. Cutting through it was a team effort. With the chest opened, we did not see the heart at first. It was cloaked by the fleshy shroud of the lungs. For all its outward symmetry, the human body is not symmetric. The left lung, for example, has only two lobes, unlike its tri-lobed counterpart on the other side. (The left lung's middle lobe atrophies during fetal development because the heart gobbles up its space.) Both of my cadaver's lungs were speckled with black: smoker's tar, I assumed, or perhaps just a remnant of city living. They felt like a waterlogged sponge, but when you squeezed them, no fluid seeped out. The cartilaginous airways were hard but pliable, like the end of a chicken bone.

My cadaver's heart was about the size of two hands clasped together in prayer, filling most of the mid-chest cavity from the breastbone to the spine and down to the diaphragm, the muscular drape that separates the chest from the abdomen. (Every time you take a breath, the beating heart, resting on the diaphragm, translates slightly downward.) The heart had the shape of a truncated ellipsoid, like a squat volcano tipped on its side. Its muscle—the myocardium—was stiff. Cardiac muscle utilizes energy to *relax*, not contract, so at death my cadaver's heart went into a state of rigor mortis. The atria, the upper collecting chambers, sat behind the ventricles, the muscular pumping chambers. The right ventricle sat most forward in the chest. It was crescent shaped, its muscle fibers running circumferentially around its exterior. Our professor told us that if ever, as doctors, we had to insert a needle into a patient's chest to drain fluid, the right ventricle is the first chamber we would hit.

A few snips and we released the heart from its beige scaffolding. A lab mate placed it on the cadaver's forearm. "This guy really wears his heart on his sleeve," he said. Gripping the organ like a Rubik's Cube, I poked my fingers into the thin-walled central veins. It was hard not to lapse into thinking that it was just a piece of meat, a rubberized toy. The left ventricle had thick walls, a sign of high blood pressure. The inside of the right ventricle was a dense morass of fibers. Maybe there were stories written in that mossy tangle, but I didn't see any. By the time we'd cleaved all the chambers open—storing the heart between sessions in a circular aluminum pan, like the kind used for baking pies—it had the color and texture of cooked beef.

Until then, it had been a mystery exactly how our cadaver had died. His ribs were just a bundle of sticks—thin and worn—so some in our group assumed he'd succumbed to one of the diseases that waste and ravage the body, such as tuberculosis or cancer. But when we finally dissected his heart, the answer was revealed. The aorta, the main artery that carries blood from the heart to the body, was marbled with a massive amount of hard, cholesterol-laden plaque. When we sliced open the left coronary artery, grit pushed back against the scalpel. Inside the artery was a long dark brown clot where an atherosclerotic plaque had ruptured. Blood-clotting platelets had surged like minnows to the site of injury, clumping together to form a thrombosis that blocked the artery, causing a heart attack and tissue death.* This was the mechanism that probably killed my

---

*Unlike the cells of lesser organs such as the liver, heart cells do not regenerate in large amounts. When they die, they are gobbled up by cells called macrophages and replaced by scar tissue.

grandfather, too (and, I worried, would eventually claim another of the Jauhar men). Baked into those coarse arterial impurities, I couldn't help but think, were my cadaver's failures and sorrows.

With the chest open, we were reminded once again of the basic scheme that sustains all mammal life. Deoxygenated blood passes from the right atrium through a one-way valve, the tricuspid, into the right ventricle, which pumps the blood into the lungs. Oxygen-rich blood returns from the lungs to fill the left atrium. The blood then passes through another valve, the mitral (so named because it resembles a bishop's miter, or headdress), into the left ventricle, from which it is pumped through the aorta and to the rest of the body. The blood eventually collects in two great veins, the inferior and superior venae cavae, which return it to the right atrium, where it again passes through the tricuspid valve into the right ventricle, to begin the cycle again.

This system, fundamental to all mammals, was not discovered until the early seventeenth century. For most of human history, the biological function of the heart was a mystery. Ten thousand years ago, Cro-Magnon hunters in Europe knew about the heart—they engraved curlicue pictures of it on the walls of caves—but they had no clue about what it did. Seven millennia later, the ancient Egyptians devised surprisingly prescient theories about the heart's purpose. They believed the heart was where the soul resided, of course, but a classic document, the Ebers Papyrus, also described the heart as the center of the blood supply, with vessels directed toward the major organs. "The actions of the arms, the movement of the legs, the motion of every other member is done according to the orders of the heart that has conceived them," the paper reads. Three thousand years later, the ancient Greeks had a mostly symbolic understanding of the heart. They believed the heart's central location in the body meant that it was the center of life and morality. Plato also proposed that the heart was a sentry—the *thymos*, the highest part of the mortal soul—through which blood

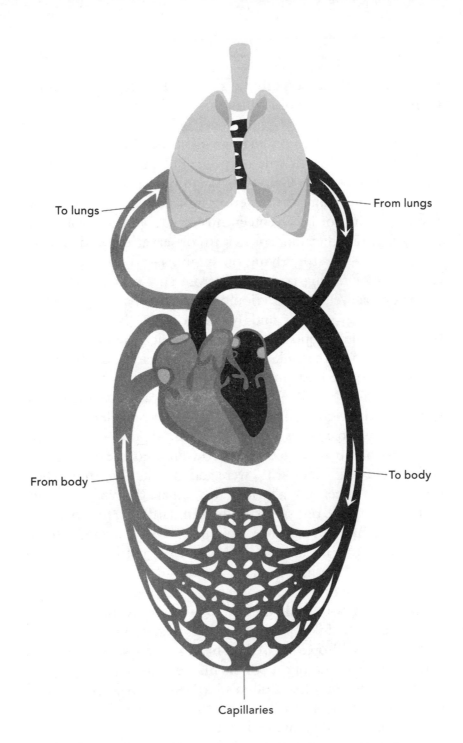

To lungs

From lungs

From body

To body

Capillaries

Circulation scheme in mammals (Created by Liam Eisenberg, Koyo Designs)

rushes to warn that something is amiss. In fact, this remains a more or less accurate description of the onset of the fight-or-flight response.

The Greeks relied on analogy—on metaphors—to try to understand the heart's true purpose. But their fanciful speculation gave way when Galen, physician of the Roman emperor Marcus Aurelius and the towering figure in Western medicine from the third to the seventeenth century, applied a rudimentary scientific method rooted in observation and animal dissections—but still relying on symbols—to the problem of circulation. Drawing conclusions from surgeries on wounded gladiators, as well as vivisection on an array of animals, including cats, dogs, sheep, and lynx—human dissections were banned—Galen proposed a scheme in which the liver converts food into blood that, like water in an irrigation ditch, travels one way into the body to be absorbed and disappear, never to be used again. In Galen's scheme, blood was sucked from the liver into the right ventricle and passed to the left ventricle through invisible pores in the wall—the septum—separating the two chambers. Once the blood entered the left ventricle, he believed "vital spirits" were added to it. The left ventricle then generated heat like a furnace to circulate the blood through fleshy pipes to the rest of the body. "In hardness, tension, general strength, and resistance to injury," Galen wrote, "the fibers of the heart far surpass all others, for no other instrument performs such continuous, hard work."

Galen's theories were accepted as the final word on cardiovascular—indeed all human—anatomy in the West. Through the Middle Ages, his writings were scripture, immune to questioning. People focused on his conclusions, not the (often scant) observations upon which his conclusions were based. Though his reasoning was often spurious and analogical—water irrigating fields, a furnace heating pipes—the scientific method, careful measurement supporting or disproving falsifiable propositions, had not yet taken hold. When observations were made that did not concur with Galenism, they were marginalized and discounted.

A more advanced understanding of the heart probably existed in Persia, where the physician Ibn al-Nafis wrote his *Commentary on Anatomy* in 1242. Ibn al-Nafis was born in Syria and received his medical education in Damascus, before moving to Cairo. In *Commentary*, one of the pinnacles of the "golden age of Islamic medicine," Ibn al-Nafis wrote that the ventricles receive nourishment from coronary vessels—not, as Galen had claimed, from blood deposited inside their chambers—and that the pulse is due to the force of cardiac contraction, not, as Galen contended, because of innate arterial contractility. Perhaps most important, Ibn al-Nafis asserted that there are no pores in the wall between the two ventricles. "There is no passage between these two cavities; for the substance of the heart is solid in this region and has neither a visible passage, as was thought by some persons, nor an invisible one which could have permitted the transmission of blood, as was alleged by Galen."

However, despite these essentially correct insights, Ibn al-Nafis's tome was unavailable in Europe and was mostly forgotten until a copy of it was discovered by a graduate student in the Prussian State Library in 1924. And so the workings of the heart remained a mystery in the West, "more deeply hidden than the step of the black ant on black rock in the black of night," as al-Ghazali, the Islamic mystic, declared.

Fortunately, the prescientific vitalism that dominated European thought gave way to the Renaissance and a greater commitment to investigation and reason. Perhaps no thinker of this period did more to advance knowledge of the heart than Leonardo da Vinci, who considered it "an admirable instrument invented by the Supreme Being." Among hundreds of Leonardo's anatomical illustrations, a great many are devoted to the cardiovascular system. His earliest studies were on pigs and oxen, but he also dissected human cadavers—about thirty in all, from infants to centenarians—that he collected from hospitals in Florence and Rome. Leonardo, like his predecessors, used natural phenomena and analogies to elucidate the workings of the heart. For example, he observed that water flowing against the banks of a river contributes to a river's tortuous meanderings, and relying on this metaphor, he hypothesized that a similar thing happened with blood vessels. Leonardo constructed glass models of the aorta and the aortic valve to investigate the dynamics of blood flow using dyed water.* His dissections also provided insights into vascular disease. "The artery and the vein acquire so great a thickness of skin that it contracts the passage of the blood," he wrote in a more or less accurate description of atherosclerotic plaque obstructing blood flow. However, the concept of a continuous, unceasing circulation eluded him.

Before a century had passed, raucous crowds were gathering at the University of Padua for public dissections. It was here—the center of European anatomy, where the world's first anatomical theater housed galleries for spectators—that perhaps history's greatest surgeon, Andreas Vesalius, worked. Vesalius's portrait hung prominently in our anatomy lab in St. Louis, his watchful eyes scrutinizing our dissections like a high priest's. The son of an apothecary, Vesalius was dissecting rats and dogs as a teen. As an academic, he performed his investigations on corpses stolen from graves and charnel houses outside Padua. He snuck them home inside his coat and stored them (unpreserved) for weeks in his apartment. A friendly criminal judge also gave Vesalius access to the gallows and even scheduled executions at times convenient to the anatomist. In *De humani corporis fabrica* (*The Fabric of the Human Body*), published in 1543 and perhaps the most venerated anatomy textbook ever written, Vesalius corrected many of Galen's mistakes

*The importance of turbulent flow for closing the aortic valve, an idea originated by Leonardo, has been confirmed only in the past decade.

about the heart, especially his claim of a porous septum between the left and the right ventricles. Vesalius rightly deduced that to get to the left side of the heart, blood must pass through the lungs. However, he also reinforced some of Galen's erroneous conclusions, such as that blood is produced by the liver and consumed in the body and that the heart is a furnace.

It wasn't until William Harvey, the brilliant English anatomist who studied at Padua in his early twenties, that Galen's theory of circulation was fully upended. Harvey was born in Kent, England, in 1578 and completed his degree in arts at Cambridge when he was nineteen. He then transferred to the University of Padua to study medicine. Although Harvey discovered the mechanism of circulation in 1615, he waited thirteen years before publishing his results. He feared for his safety; challenging Galenic dogma was considered sacrilegious. He might have been worried that he'd suffer the same fate as Michael Servetus, a theologian who was burned at the stake in Geneva at the age of forty-two, in part for promoting the idea that blood passes through the lungs. "What remains

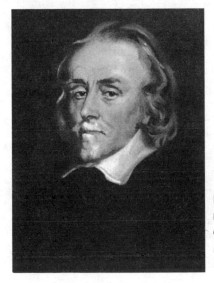

Portrait of William Harvey (From Domenico Ribatti, "William Harvey and the Discovery of the Circulation of the Blood," *Journal of Angiogenesis Research* 1 [2009]: 3)

to be said upon the quantity and source of the blood which thus passes," Harvey wrote, "is of a character so novel and unheard-of that I not only fear injury to myself from the envy of a few, but I tremble lest I have mankind at large for my enemies."*

In *De motu cordis*, a seventy-two-page monograph written in Latin and published in 1628, when Harvey was fifty, Harvey set as his task "to look a little more deeply into the matter [of circulation]; to contemplate the movements of the arteries and of the heart not only in man, but also in other animals." At first, he wrote, "I found the task so truly arduous . . . that I was almost tempted to think . . . that the movement of the heart was only to be comprehended by God." Harvey decided to study the hearts of fish and frogs, whose contractions were slow enough to be analyzed. He also experimented on live and dead humans. In a simple but ingenious experiment, Harvey tied off a human arm with cloth, cutting off blood flow. He then relaxed the tourniquet so that arterial blood at higher pressure could pass but venous blood could not. The arm quickly swelled, leading Harvey to infer that blood flowed down arteries and drained through invisible connections into veins before returning to the heart. The nature of these connections—today we would call them capillaries—was a puzzle that Harvey never solved.† However, it did not deter him from his fundamental conclusions: that the heart is a pump, and that blood circulates

---

*In his later years, Harvey reportedly said to a friend, "You know very well the storm my previous research caused. It is often better to grow wise in private at home, than to publish what you have amassed with infinite labor, to stir up storms that may rob you of peace and quiet for the rest of your days."

†Capillaries were discovered three decades later, in 1661, when Marcello Malpighi looked at sections of frog lung under a microscope. Malpighi referred to frogs as the "microscope of nature" because they allowed him to see structures that were not visible in larger animals. Nature is accustomed, he wrote, "to undertake its great works only after a series of attempts at lower levels, and to outline in imperfect animals the plan of perfect animals." He added, "For the unloosing of these knots I have destroyed almost the whole race of frogs."

continuously in a closed circuit from the arteries to the veins and back again.

Harvey's opus is filled with references to Galen's work, but as is so often the case in science, the student surpassed his teacher. When Harvey tied off a section of artery with two ligatures and cut it open, he discovered that there was only blood inside, not air or spirits, as Galen had claimed, or "sooty vapours," as Harvey disdainfully called them. Of the tiny holes in the ventricular septum that Galen said allow blood to pass from the right ventricle to the left, Harvey wrote, "Damme, there are no pores. It is not possible to show such."* He correctly deduced, as a few others had before him, that the flow had to be through the lungs. Harvey calculated that if the average adult heart expels two ounces of blood per beat (roughly true) at seventy-two beats per minute, the liver would have to produce five hundred pounds of blood from food *per hour* if blood were consumed as a nutrient, an obvious impossibility. Therefore, in Harvey's scheme, blood was the transport vehicle for nourishment, not the nourishment itself. Like Galen and the natural philosophers before him, Harvey relied on metaphorical reasoning. "The heart is the center of life, the sun of the Microcosm, as the sun itself might be called the heart of the world," he wrote. But Harvey's metaphors—the circular motion of planets, the recycling of water on earth—were better suited for the problem of circulation.†

---

*Through experiments, Harvey proved that when the pulmonary artery is ligated and the right ventricle is injected with water, no fluid crosses the septum into the left ventricle.

†Harvey's analogies extended to the body politic. He wrote to King Charles I in the preface to *De motu cordis*, "What I have here written of the motions of the heart I am the more emboldened to present to your Majesty, according to the custom of the present age, because almost all things human are done after human examples, and many things in a King are after the pattern of the heart. The knowledge of his heart, therefore, will not be useless to a Prince, as embracing a kind of Divine example of his functions—and it has still been usual with men to compare small things with great. Here, at all events, best of Princes, placed as you are on

Though Harvey solved a problem that had vexed philosophers for millennia, perhaps his greatest contribution was in demonstrating the power of experiment to confirm or reject hypotheses. In his Harveian Oration in 1906, Sir William Osler, the Canadian physician, said of *De motu cordis*, "At last came the age of the hand—the thinking, devising, planning hand, the hand as an instrument of the mind, now reintroduced into the world in a modest little monograph from which we may date the beginning of experimental medicine." However, despite his fundamental discoveries, Harvey never understood the purpose of circulation. He figured out the *how* of circulation but not the *why*. In his book he wrote that blood "returns to its source, the heart, the inner temple of the body, to recover its virtue." But what was that "virtue"? And why was there a difference in color between crimson venous and cherry arterial blood? The answers to these two questions are of course the same. But Harvey and his followers were unaware of the oxygen-carrying function of red blood cells—indeed, ignorant of oxygen itself. Those discoveries would have to wait a hundred years.

Today we know that the right ventricle pumps blood to the lungs, where oxygen is added via microscopic air sacs to red blood cells in the lung's capillaries. From the lungs, oxygen-rich blood passes through the pulmonary veins to the left heart, which pumps it through the aorta and through smaller and smaller arteries to the rest of the body to meet the body's metabolic demands. Blood that has delivered its oxygen drains through capillaries into veins and finally into the superior and inferior venae cavae to return to the right heart to begin the cycle anew. Laid end to end, the vast network of capillaries in the human body would encircle the globe. Their total cross-sectional area would cover several football fields. Although the

---

the pinnacle of human affairs, you may at once contemplate the prime mover in the body of man, and the emblem of your own sovereign power."

pressure in the veins is low, the pressure in the right heart is even lower, and this provides the necessary push to drive blood back to its pump.

The muscular ventricles pump blood by contracting their fibers in response to electrical stimulation. Each muscle fiber is composed of protein filaments that are stimulated by electrical current to slide past one another, thus allowing the organ to squeeze and then relax, emptying and filling, in repetitive fashion, billions of times over the lifetime of the animal. The pressure the heart generates is the highest of all the organs, propelling blood through an immense array of arteries that get smaller and smaller, branching like twigs to nourish every cell in the body.

Blood circulates in one direction only. Backflow is prevented through one-way valves. When a valve does not close properly, it allows blood to flow in the opposite direction, a useless expenditure of energy. If a valve does not properly open, it limits the flow forward. In both cases, circulation is impaired. In an indelible pearl of wisdom, our anatomy professor told us that a cardiac anomaly can sometimes cancel another anomaly, if only incompletely. For instance, if a valve does not open, blood must find a path around the obstruction. Such a detour—a hole between chambers, for example, or an anomalous connection— can have devastating consequences in an otherwise normal heart, but in a diseased heart it may actually attenuate the pathology. In the human heart, he said, two wrongs can make an imperfect right.

•

At the end of that first semester of medical school, on a freezing January evening, we honored a school tradition and held a memorial service for our cadavers on the twelfth floor of the hospital. (Their remains were going to be cremated afterward.) Four long rows of wooden chairs were filled. Lights were dimmed, and candles were lit; the ceremony was grave and ritualistic, befitting the solemn occasion. People stepped up to recite poems they'd written. A chaplain spoke. A few students sang songs or performed on guitar. Our professor, now stripped of latex gloves and blue scrubs and wearing a crisp navy suit, walked up to the podium to deliver a eulogy. "Who were your donors?" he asked us again. Had we taken the time to think about the lives they might have led? By then, we had dissected most of them away, and yet their last act would live on in each of us. It was our responsibility, he said, to ensure their gift—the ultimate gift—had been worthwhile.

A part of me wanted to go up and tell the narrative I'd dreamed up about my cadaver. He had come to America for graduate school, one of the brave first in a wave of South Asian immigrants after World War II. He had probably never set foot outside the country. He had only known his gray house in Punjab, with the white railing on the rooftop, and the congested streets where farm animals roamed amid noxious vapors of dung and exhaust. When he was accepted to an American university, his father surely regretted that he'd pushed his son into demanding an American education. He'll get lost, his father thought, and won't remember how to come home. Or worse, he thought, he won't want to.

I would have liked to tell my fellow students a story about an immigrant with a broken heart. It would have been in keeping with the atmosphere that evening. But I had a change of heart and remained seated.

At twenty-seven years old, I had been introduced to a man with no name. I had handled his body, cut it apart, and put it back together again. From that point on, I thought, every careless mistake I might make in the hospital would be a slap in his face, every success a tribute to him, my first patient. He had given himself freely—wholeheartedly—and now I had to give him back and leave him to restful peace.

PART II

Machine

3

Clutch

Man cannot live with a broken heart.
  —Gabriele Falloppio, sixteenth-century anatomist

From the beginning of my cardiology fellowship, there was
never really any doubt about how we were supposed to think
about the heart. Despite its metaphors, the heart in disease was
best understood as a complicated pump. At orientation, on
July 1, 2001, a dozen of us white-coated fellows scattered into
a large auditorium at Bellevue Hospital in New York City to
listen to the faculty tell us about the myriad procedures we were
going to learn that year. Isaac Abramson, the chief of echocardiography, boasted of the many applications of cardiac ultrasound, which allowed cardiologists to make diagnoses that had
once required bodily invasion. Sporting a dusty tweed jacket,
Abramson was an old-school Israeli curmudgeon, grumpy and
growly for even that part of the world. He had basically pioneered an important advance in echocardiography in the 1970s
and had spent the intervening years gathering laurels. He once
said to me, "Sam, I want the fellows to feel they are so unim-
portant that I cannot be bothered to even remember their
names." Abramson had certain tenets, nuggets of wisdom, and

on that day he dispensed one of his favorites: "Everything depends on pressure differences." He would encourage us to think about blood flow, lung congestion, and even human affairs in those terms.

Sitting next to him were his associates: David Asch, the straitlaced assistant echo chief, who thought almost as much of himself as Abramson did because he worked with the master, basking in reflected glory, which in his mind made him a bit great, too; Cindy Feldman, the only woman in the group, whose wicked humor and crazy blue eyeliner belied her astonishing clinical competence; and Richard Belkin, the anal-retentive associate fellowship director, who cared about the fellows only insofar as we reflected on him and his job performance.

The electrophysiologists sat two rows behind. The chief, Robert Dresner, an electrical presence himself—more rabbi than physician—spoke of the wonders of radio-frequency ablations, in which radiation-emitting catheters were threaded through veins into the heart to cure many common rhythm disturbances. Seated next to him was his assistant, Mitch Shapiro, a sharp and avowedly vulgar man with a neatly trimmed goatee, faintly canine in appearance, who took pride in saying outrageous things in the name of candor. ("What do you mean, 'in my heart'? 'In my fucking heart' won't hold up in a court of law.") In attitude and deportment, Shapiro was a boxer dog. Their colleague, Jim Harwood, the token researcher, was sitting off to the side, probably thinking about the cellular ion channel research he'd been muttering about for years that nobody—perhaps including Harwood himself—understood.

Sid Fuchs, the cardiac catheterization chief, had the last word. Fuchs was a weird guy; word around the hospital was that his studio apartment was occupied by a massive train set. With arched eyebrows over narrow-set eyes, Fuchs resembled a bearded Art Carney. "Don't mind my colleagues," he told us fellows after everyone had said his or her piece. "In the end, cardiology is mostly a problem of plumbing."

Whatever their idiosyncrasies, I looked up to these doctors. I wasn't sure how much I had in common with them, but essentially I knew I wanted to be like them. Understanding how and why my grandfather had died, and what implications his premature death had for my father, my siblings, and me, was fundamentally intertwined with my decision to train in cardiology. The field was also fast-paced and exciting, as if flowing out of the steady beating of the heart itself. Just as important, the considerable effort of cardiology practice was balanced by tangible rewards for patients. Unlike neurologists, master diagnosticians who had depressingly little to offer their patients, cardiologists had been at the forefront of technological innovation over the past half century. This golden period had witnessed a hailstorm of life-prolonging advances, including coronary bypass surgery, coronary stents, and implantable pacemakers and defibrillators. The dazzling technological complexity of the field was reflected in the apprehension most doctors had in managing heart disease. The same doctor who felt comfortable treating diabetes, kidney failure, or anemia would consult a cardiologist for even a mildly abnormal electrocardiogram (EKG). The heart can kill quickly, without warning, faster than any organ, which inspired fear in even the most seasoned doctor. And so a fellowship in cardiology was like entering an exclusive club, a club that incredibly had decided to take me as a member.

Of course, I was nervous. Every new doctor should be. Cardiologists specialize in emergencies. The culture is pressurized. In neuroscience, there is the concept of the reflex arc, in which a threatening stimulus can effect a response without passing through the conscious brain—for example, when you see the taillight flash red on the car speeding in front of you and your foot automatically moves to the brake pedal. I was afraid that now, as a cardiologist in training, I would have to acquire a new reflex arc.

For the first few months of my fellowship, that summer of

2001, I spent a portion of every call night pacing back and forth in my living room, my armpits moist—and not just because of the broken air-conditioning—trying to memorize algorithms for treating the major cardiac emergencies; I might as well have been in the hospital. I often thought back to an experience I'd had in medical school. It happened during my first clinical clerkship in internal medicine at the beginning of my third year in St. Louis. I was working with a star resident of the internal medicine program. David, cardiology bound, was confident, competent, and quick. He thrived under pressure.

One afternoon, my team was called to the cardiac care unit (CCU). A patient, James Abbott, had just been admitted with excruciating chest pain that had started a few hours earlier. He was in his early fifties, extensively tattooed, just the sort of tough I wouldn't want to meet alone in a parking lot at night, but right then he was whimpering. He kept stroking his sternum up and down, as if trying to rub the pain away. It was obvious that he was having a heart attack. He had all the classic risk factors: hypertension, high cholesterol, a history of cigarette smoking. His electrocardiogram and blood tests showed characteristic signs of low blood flow to the heart muscle. I don't recall our examining him, but for this most common type of cardiac emergency, there is little diagnostic role for the physical exam.

A few hours later, we were paged back to the CCU. Abbott was now writhing in pain, and his blood pressure was dropping. David had a nurse get another EKG. He ordered an intern to prepare to insert a catheter into Abbott's radial artery. Then he asked for an intubation tray to put him on a ventilator. "Check his blood pressure," he told me.

As a medical student, I had measured blood pressure only a few times, mostly in my classmates. I carefully wrapped the cuff around Abbott's left arm and inflated it. Then I let the pressure out slowly, listening with my stethoscope at the bend of his arm. "One hundred over sixty," I called out.

"Check the other arm," David said. By then he was scrubbing Abbott's arm with iodine soap in preparation for an arterial line. More people arrived, attracted by the commotion. I wrapped the cuff around the right arm and quickly inflated it, but when I let out the pressure, I heard nothing. Must be doing something wrong, I thought. I tried again while people jostled me, with the same result. Must be the noise, I told myself, so I shrugged and let it go. For a moment I thought to ask David to check the pressure himself, but he was busy doing more important things. So I stepped aside to give others access, before being quickly pushed to the fringe.

The next morning, David caught me before rounds. His face was pale. "That guy had an aortic dissection," he said. A CT scan had revealed a corkscrew-like tear from the abdominal aorta all the way back to the heart. "The night resident picked it up," he said. "He noticed there was a pulse deficit between the arms. No pressure on the right."

I listened in silence. A pulse deficit is a classic sign of aortic dissection, but in the hubbub of the previous afternoon I had somehow ignored it. I thought about telling David about the blood pressure measurement I had taken, but I didn't. Abbott's dissection was by now far advanced, and surgeons who had been consulted said he would not survive an operation. He died eight hours later.

For weeks I couldn't get over the idea that I was somehow responsible for Abbott's death. If we had caught the dissection the previous day, there was a chance at least that he could have been saved. I eventually managed to convince myself that the death wasn't entirely my fault. But that didn't make me any less afraid of cardiac patients.

•

As a first-year cardiology fellow, the main reason you'd get called in the middle of the night was to perform an echocardiogram, using an ultrasound probe to take pictures of the heart, which residents were not trained to do. There were many possible reasons to do an echo urgently, but the most common was to check for cardiac tamponade: fluid accumulating in the pericardium, the sac around the heart, thus squeezing the heart and hindering its ability to fill with blood. Cardiac tamponade is life threatening; rapid collection of pericardial fluid or blood can quickly put the heart into a standstill. Without proper cardiac filling and emptying, blood flow and pressure plummet and a person goes into shock. (Christ, nailed to the cross, likely succumbed to tamponade after receiving a laceration to his heart by the lance of a Roman soldier.)

In 1761, Giovanni Battista Morgagni, an Italian anatomist, spoke of the dangers of cardiac compression from hemorrhage into the pericardium. He noted that puncture of a coronary artery on the external surface of the heart could cause blood to pour into the pericardial sac, squeezing all chambers. How serious the compromise depends on how quickly the fluid accumulates. The pericardium is like a balloon. When you blow up a balloon, you must generate enough pressure to overcome the tension of the rubber. It gets easier the second time because the rubber has already been stretched. Similarly, slow accumulation of fluid stretches the pericardial membrane, making it thin and compliant and keeping the pressure inside the space low. Rapid filling, on the other hand, before the pericardium has been stretched, can result in a quick rise in pericardial pressure that can push on and collapse the heart's chambers, thus compromising blood flow. At that point, you would have to put a needle through the chest and into the pericardial sac to drain the fluid, which I had never done.* As I paced the living room on those summer nights in 2001, it occurred to me that there was a curious analogy between tamponade and my first nights on call.

---

*Tamponade is a last-drop phenomenon: a small amount of extra fluid in the pericardium can cause the blood pressure to plummet. Fortunately, it is also a first-drop phenomenon: extracting even a small amount of fluid can restore blood flow and life.

I knew that my tolerance for emergencies would develop. I knew that a slow accumulation of experience would eventually deliver confidence and courage. But until it did, I was terrified that a patient I was responsible for would crash and burn.

Senior fellows had warned us that surgeons would request echos on flimsy grounds. A post-op patient might have a slight decrease in blood pressure, and they'd want an echo to rule out tamponade. A patient might have a slight increase in his liver enzymes, and the surgical fellow would say it was because of hepatic vein congestion—unlikely!—and want to rule out tamponade. Sometimes you'd ask for a patient's vital signs, and it would turn out the patient had normal heart rate and blood pressure, and the surgical fellow—on call and under the gun himself—would admit he was just being cautious. In that case, senior fellows urged us to push back, question, cajole—"Dude, can't this wait until morning?"—anything short of outright refusal, which could get you fired.

Most nights just the expectation of the pager going off was enough to keep me awake, anxiously rubbing my feet together in bed, waiting for the inevitable call. And just when my consciousness would begin to fade in the pale darkness, the piercing ring. You'd never know how long the beeper had been going off, just that the night had finally begun. I'd pull myself up, being careful not to wake up my wife, Sonia, quickly push the jigsaw pieces of my awareness back together, and then tiptoe to the living room to answer the call.

The first page I ever got was to do an echo on a woman with breast cancer who had become acutely short of breath. I started off by challenging the request—what were the patient's vitals, how long had her pressure been low—but something about the surgical fellow's tone told me to shut up and just go in. So I threw on my scrubs; grabbed my stethoscope; stuffed a $20 bill, a ballpoint pen, and my hospital ID into my vest pocket; and hurried down to the street to catch a yellow cab going downtown.

Three o'clock in the morning in my neighborhood was when

the rats came out, and the mere threat of one of those mon-
sters darting out from sidewalk garbage was enough to make
me stand in the middle of the empty street. The storefronts
were mostly unlit, save for a few randomly glowing windows. A
speeding taxi quickly came to a screeching halt to let me in. We
took a roller-coaster ride down the FDR Drive, under bridges
and through tunnels, the concrete walls rushing at me as shad-
ows of the metropolis reflected off the dashboard like colonies
on an agar plate. In the distance you could see the high-rises on
Roosevelt Island dotted with lights, like a yellow pox, and beyond them the Brooklyn Bridge and the smokestacks of the
Lower East Side. In my mind, I went through the different
ultrasound views I'd have to show Dr. Abramson the following
morning. Did I remember how to adjust the frequency filters
and sweep speed? Abramson, the echo chief, could be tough.
His merciless interrogation at an early-morning conference
had already made a first-year fellow faint and drop to the floor.

The driver let me off in the lot behind Bellevue. Here the
rats were even bigger, moving almost randomly, like leaves propelled by gusts of wind. The hospital rose up to the cloudless
sky like some sort of gothic hotel. Looking up at the building,
I could only imagine what life-or-death drama was awaiting me.
At the entrance, young hipsters with black leather jackets and
lip rings were sprawled on the sidewalk. In the lobby, the air
was stale, slightly smoky. I quickly flashed my ID badge to the
burly security guard. Then I jogged over to the echo lab on the
second floor to grab a bottle of Aquasonic gel and the bulky
Siemens machine, which I steered down narrow desolate corridors to the surgical intensive care unit.

Three thirty in the morning is a strange time to be awake,
the nexus between night and day, when things are supposed to
move slowly and trying to speed them up seems almost obscene.
When I pushed through the double doors of the surgical unit,
it was like entering a casino, with flashing lights, chiming
bells, and its share of lost souls. Family members were loitering

in the hallways or sitting at bedsides, keeping vigil. The faintly pleasant smell of disinfectant and talcum powder wafted through the corridors. I poked my head into the conference room looking for the surgical fellow. The room was littered with printouts, X-rays, and the detritus of the previous evening's meal. No fellow. I plodded to the nursing station, where a young woman was inputting data into a computer. Without looking up, she pointed to a room at the corner of the unit.

I maneuvered my echo machine into the tiny space between the patient's bed and the wailing monitor. The woman had a willful look, as if she were trying not to appear panicked, even though she obviously was. Short wispy hair stood up on her scalp like newly germinated grass. Her eyes darted back and forth, like a scared child's, even as she insisted that she was fine. Her blood pressure, the monitor above her bed informed me, was dirt.

The body attempts to compensate for a rapid drop in blood pressure (called shock) through a number of mechanisms. There is increased sympathetic and reduced parasympathetic activity in the autonomic nerves, speeding up the heart rate and increasing cardiac output. Salt and water are reabsorbed in the kidneys. Small peripheral arteries constrict to shunt blood away from nonessential areas of the body, like the skin and skeletal muscles, to vital organs, such as the heart, kidneys, and brain. Gas exchange in the lungs is impaired, causing blood acids to build up and the breathing rate to increase.

All these changes seemed to be happening in my patient at once. In the jaundiced light she appeared pale, the color of bone. Her heartbeat sounded like a galloping horse. She was quiet, because she could not talk and breathe at the same time. When I applied the echo probe to her bandaged chest, where a breast tumor had been surgically removed, even I could tell that a massive amount of blood had accumulated in the pericardial sac. The heart looked like a small animal confined to a tiny pool, like one of Richter's rats stuck in a swimming jar, struggling to get free. The right ventricle was compressed like a pancake. It was almost a relief to finally see the thing I'd feared and face it. I ran out to tell the surgical fellow, and almost immediately he was in a sterile gown, and I was being asked to step to one side, out of the way but still close enough to hold the echo probe in place to guide the drainage needle via ultrasound.

A nurse threw a blanket over the patient. The fellow tore open a surgical kit. The woman had stopped moving under the drape. She was either being extremely cooperative or sinking into shock. After numbing the skin below the breastbone with lidocaine anesthetic, the fellow pierced it with a six-inch-long needle, directing the tip, with the aid of my ultrasound, directly at the heart. The right ventricle sits most anterior in the chest, protected only by the pericardium and a thin layer of fat. I remembered what our anatomy professor had told us: if we ever had to push a needle through the chest wall, the right ventricle is the first structure we would hit. On the echo screen the needle tip entered the pericardium, scattering the ultrasound into a white halo, like a white sun in a hazy black sea. The barrel of the syringe was pulled back, and maroon-colored fluid burst into the plastic column. The fellow removed the syringe from the needle, and the bloody effusion trickled out. Then he pushed a catheter through the barrel of the needle, attached it to a drainage bag, and quickly stitched it in. Within minutes, the drape was off, and as best I could tell, the patient had regained her color. Her blood pressure was now almost normal as bloody cancerous fluid drained into the bag.

A few minutes of delay, arguing with the surgical fellow or waiting longer for a cab, and the woman would surely have died. The surgical fellow, a pleasant Indian man, was grateful. It turned out that he himself had had heart surgery as a child (he pulled down the V-neck of his scrubs to show me the pasty, indistinct scar at the top of the breastbone). We got along well after that night, a kinship born, as is common in a teaching hospital, out of facing a harrowing experience together. It was my first time confronting a live, beating heart in an emergency. And for a few more months, at least, I never argued another echo request.

•

Inge Edler, a cardiologist, and Carl Hellmuth Hertz, a physicist, invented echocardiography at the University of Lund in Sweden in the early 1950s. They went to shipyards to study sonar, making the conceptual leap that if you can use ultrasound to see a ship five hundred meters away, maybe you can use it to see the heart, too, if only you could change the depth of penetration. They made a prototype probe and put it on Edler's chest. They did not know what they were seeing at first, but they could tell it was a beating heart. In 1954, they published the first paper on cardiac ultrasound, titled "The Use of Ultrasonic Reflectoscope for the Continuous Recording of the Movements of Heart Walls." In the mid-1960s, Harvey Feigenbaum first used ultrasound to study pericardial fluid accumulations. Soon, echocardiography was widely employed to rapidly localize a fluid collection and help surgeons direct their drainage needles. Ultrasound made treating cardiac tamponade almost protocol. Indeed, after a few months of my fellowship, tamponade did not seem like such a big deal.

But tamponade was a very big deal in early operating theaters, where cardiac injuries loomed especially large. And it was the driving force on a revolutionary summer day in 1893, when Dr. Daniel Hale Williams, a surgeon at Provident Hospital in Chicago, drained a traumatic pericardial effusion in what was then believed to be the first open-heart surgery. The patient, twenty-four-year-old James Cornish, had been stabbed with a knife in the chest in a saloon scuffle. He was bleeding profusely when he was dropped off at the hospital by a horse-drawn ambulance. With no diagnostic equipment other than a stethoscope—X-rays would not be discovered for another two years—Williams examined him. The stab wound was slightly to the left of the breastbone and directly over the right ventricle.

Initially, he thought it was superficial, but when Cornish started to exhibit lethargy, listlessness, and low blood pressure—signs of tamponade and shock—Williams knew he had to act.

Nothing in Williams's hardscrabble life could have predicted this epoch-making moment. His father, a barber, died of tuberculosis when Williams was only ten. He was sent to live with family friends in Baltimore. Largely self-taught, he took up odd jobs, becoming a shoemaker's apprentice, then a barber and a guitar player on lake boats, before deciding to pursue medicine. He ended up in Chicago, working as a surgical apprentice and eventually completing his training at Chicago Medical College (later, Northwestern University Medical School). He set up his own practice on the South Side, working as a doctor in an orphanage and becoming the first black surgeon to work for the city's railway system. Williams, whose ancestors were slaves, worked with the Equal Rights League, a black civil rights organization that was active during Reconstruction and beyond. In 1891, he founded Provident Hospital, the nation's first racially integrated facility for young black doctors and nurses, in a three-story redbrick house in Cook County. The facility, championed by the social reformer Frederick Douglass, gave blacks in Chicago another place, besides overcrowded charity hospitals, to receive care.

Until that summer day in 1893, surgery had scarcely ever been attempted on a live human heart.* Though it is difficult to fathom today, when invasive cardiac treatments are at the forefront of medicine, the heart was essentially off-limits to doctors until almost the beginning of the twentieth century. All major human organs, including the brain, had been operated on, but the heart stood apart, encased in historical and cultural pro-

---

*There are reports of sporadic attempts on the battlefield, which were likely unsuccessful. Henry Dalton, a little-known St. Louis surgeon, is often credited with the first suture of the pericardium of a stabbing victim in 1891, but his achievement was not widely reported.

hibitions much thicker than its membranous pericardium. Heart surgery had been performed on animals, and in 1651, William Harvey himself had catheterized the inferior vena cava in a human cadaver, but suturing the dancing organ in a live person was considered beyond the realm of the possible. "The heart alone of all the viscera cannot withstand injury," Aristotle wrote, because it was believed to be impossible to mend a heart wound. Filled with blood, the heart bleeds quickly. There seemed to be no way to isolate it from the bloodstream to allow for careful stitching. Galen himself noted that heart wounds in gladiators were always fatal. "When a perforation penetrated one of the cardiac ventricles," he wrote, "they died on the spot, mainly by blood loss, and even faster if the left ventricle was injured." Therefore, as late as the early nineteenth century, the prescribed treatment for cardiac wounds leading to fluid accumulation and tamponade was absolute quiet and the application of leeches. Not surprising, then, that more than 90 percent of patients died.* But despite this awful mortality rate, Theodor Billroth, a distinguished Viennese professor and surgeon, still wrote in 1875 that "[drainage] of the pericardium is an operation which, in my opinion, approaches very closely to that kind of intervention which some surgeons would term a prostitution of the surgical act and other madness." However, he added, "further generations may think differently."

Billroth did not have to wait a generation. Already, by the late nineteenth century, proscriptions against heart surgery were being eased. In 1881, at the Anatomical and Surgical Society of Brooklyn, the surgeon John Bingham Roberts announced that "the time may possibly come when wounds of the heart itself will be treated by pericardial incision to allow extraction of clots and perhaps to suture the cardiac muscle." In 1882, M. Block, a German doctor, revealed that he had made and stitched

*In 1868, Georg Fischer analyzed 452 cases of heart wounds and found the survival rate to be only 10 percent.

puncture wounds in the hearts of rabbits, who had survived. He suggested similar techniques might work in humans. In New York, the surgeon Charles Albert Elsberg reported that his animal experiments "seem to show that a mammalian heart will bear a much greater amount of manipulation than has hitherto been suspected."

In their midst was Daniel Williams, a showboating surgeon who made up in boldness and technical prowess what he lacked in humility. Later in his career, when he was at Howard University, he would become famous for inviting the public into the hospital on Sunday afternoons to watch him operate—"when the Negro public had not become accustomed to Negro physicians and had not learned to have full confidence in them," as the anthropologist W. Montague Cobb noted. "Many dreaded to cross the threshold of a hospital, any hospital," Cobb added. "Dr. Williams took the boldest and most thorough-going step possible [to] combat this irrational fear. He threw open the doors of his operating room once a week to the public and said in effect, 'Come watch us work, observe conditions and see for yourselves that there is nothing to be afraid of.'"

James Cornish was no well-chosen public demonstration, though. When Williams opened his chest wound with a six-inch incision that sweltering day in 1893, he had no idea what he would find. On the inner surface of the ribs, a lacerated artery was trickling blood. Williams sutured it closed with catgut. The operating room was like a sauna; assistants wiped a similar dribble from Williams's brow. Williams was getting ready to close the chest when he noticed the knife had traveled deeper, puncturing the pericardium with a hole about one-tenth of an inch in diameter. With little time to mull over his options, he asked for more catgut and needle and stitched the pericardial wound closed, carefully timing the movement of his needle with the beating heart in a sort of surgical tango. He noted that there was also a small wound in the thin-walled right ventricle—in the heart muscle itself—but it had formed a dark clot on its surface and was no longer bleeding. Williams decided to leave it alone.

Cornish's wound re-bled after a few days, so Williams took him back to the OR to evacuate more clot. The wound eventually healed, and Cornish escaped the clutches of sepsis, the great postoperative killer in those days. On August 30, nearly two months after he was stabbed, Cornish walked out of the hospital. Apart from a few more bar fights, he went on to live a normal life, even outliving his surgeon by twelve years.

Williams's operation, we now know, was not the very first pericardial surgery. Probably three others had been performed over the previous decade, though they had not been reported widely. Williams almost certainly did not know about them, and most patients had died soon after the operations. By applying needle to pericardium in "the first successful or unsuccessful case of suture of the pericardium that has ever been recorded," as Williams himself declared, he did as much as any doctor in history to demystify the heart and advance the notion that it was a machine that could be repaired. For this he received worldwide acclaim. The fact that he was a black man living in the era of Jim Crow makes his achievement that much greater. In 1894, he moved to Washington, D.C., where he was appointed by President Grover Cleveland surgeon in chief at Freedmen's Hospital, which provided care for former slaves. He eventually moved back to Chicago, where he had an honorable (and honored) career, dying in 1931 of complications from a stroke.

Though Williams is often credited with performing the first documented open-heart surgery, he did not in fact cut into the heart. He only stitched closed the pericardium, the sac around the heart. Credit for the first myocardial stitch resulting in survival belongs to Ludwig Rehn, a German surgeon, who, on September 9, 1896, almost exactly three years after Cornish walked out of Provident Hospital, sutured a two-centimeter laceration in the right ventricle of a twenty-two-year-old Frankfurt gardener who'd been stabbed in the chest while walking in

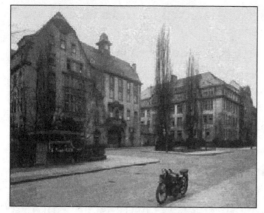

The hospital in Frankfurt, Germany, where Ludwig Rehn performed the world's first successful heart surgery (Courtesy of the *Journal of Medical Biography* 20, no. 1 [2012])

a park. The victim, Wilhelm Justus, was found by police in a state of collapse, his clothes soaked with blood. He was brought to Frankfurt State Hospital in the dark of the early morning. Though the track of the wound pointed toward the right ventricle, doctors admitted him for observation—aware, no doubt, that heart surgery conferred little benefit over prayer. But soon there were signs that blood was rapidly accumulating in his chest. Justus spiked a fever, and his respiratory rate rose to sixty-eight breaths per minute (six times faster than normal). Camphor, a stimulant, and ice bags were ordered, but Justus's condition worsened. That evening, his skin blue, pulse weak, and breathing increasingly labored, Rehn finally took him to the OR.

Born in 1849 in Allenstein, Germany, Rehn, like Williams, experienced the death of his father, a physician, when he was young and went to live with relatives. But unlike Williams, when he was presented with the opportunity to stitch a myocardial wound, he took it. He made a fourteen-centimeter incision in the space between Justus's fourth and fifth ribs along the nipple line, cut through the fifth rib, and then bent it upward, still attached to the breastbone, to create space to operate. He found an inch-long wound in the right ventricle spitting blood, spurting wildly with every contraction. "The sight of the heart beating in the opened pericardial sac was extraordinary," Rehn wrote. "Digital pressure controlled the bleeding, but my finger tended to slip off of the rapidly beating heart." He inserted a digit into the wound, then stitched the hole closed with three fine silk sutures. "It was very disquieting to see the heart pause with each pass of the needle," he wrote. But the heart soon "resumed its forceful contractions." After placement of the final stitch, the pulse was strong. Rehn turned down the rib, realigned the skin and soft tissues, and bandaged up the chest.

In that essentially pre-antiseptic era, the Grim Reaper appeared more often bearing a thermometer than a scythe. Ten days after the operation, Justus spiked a temperature of 104 degrees Fahrenheit. Pus leaked from his chest wound. He had developed sepsis. Rehn took him back to the OR to drain the infection. Fortunately, the fever quickly resolved, and Justus's condition improved. He was discharged home a week later.

Six months later, on April 22, 1897, Rehn described his operation at a surgical meeting in Berlin, where he pronounced that "the feasibility of cardiac repair no longer remains in doubt." "I trust that this case will not remain a curiosity, but rather, that the field of cardiac surgery will be further investigated," he said, adding that "many lives can be saved that were previously counted as lost." Rehn wrote a detailed account of his operation in a surgical journal. His wording was careful, even a bit defensive. Scarcely a decade earlier the great Billroth had proclaimed that "the surgeon who would attempt to suture a wound of the heart should lose the respect of his colleagues." Perhaps feeling the weight of history bearing down on him, Rehn wrote, "I was forced to operate. There was no other option open to me, with the patient lying before me, bleeding to death."

Rehn's and Williams's operations ushered in a new era in medicine in which the scalpel was finally applied to the most celebrated and elusive organ in the human body. Doctors took heed of their results. In 1899, the German surgeon Sanitatsrath Pagenstecher wrote, "I am far from wanting to make heart operations into typical procedures practiced by any physician, although efforts so far have shown very good results." On September 14, 1902, on a kitchen table under the flickering lights of two kerosene lamps in a slum shack in Montgomery, Alabama, Luther Hill became the first American surgeon to successfully suture a cardiac wound, in the left ventricle of a thirteen-year-old boy who had been stabbed five times. At a conference in 1907, Rehn reported that 120 surgeries on the heart had been performed around the world, with 40 percent of them successful, a fourfold improvement in mortality compared with the pre-surgical era. Several years later, the German surgeon Rudolf Haecker wrote, "Since ancient times, the heart has been regarded as 'noli me tangere' [but] with [heart surgery] the last organ of the human body has now fallen to the hand of the surgeon."

The dawn of heart surgery was long, however, and the full light of day would not break for several decades. Though attempts to repair almost uniformly fatal heart wounds were greeted with resigned acceptance, cutting open the organ to fix diseased valves, pitted walls, or misplaced vessels that killed slowly was still wholly rejected. The obstacles were many, but the major one was lack of time. As G. Wayne Miller writes in his authoritative book *King of Hearts*, "To open the living heart was to kill, in a river of blood that ran dry in less than a minute." To prevent such bleeding, the heart had to be isolated from the circulation and stopped before being sliced open. But stopping the heart for more than a couple of minutes would result in brain and other organ damage. How to circulate blood and oxygen after interrupting the heartbeat? This was a challenge on a scale that medicine had never encountered. Could the heart, nature's ultimate machine, be replaced by a man-made pump?

4

Dynamo

"Lemme tell you something. There's one of these doctors in Atlanta that's taken a knife and cut the human heart— the human heart," he repeated, leaning forward, "out of a man's chest and held it in his hand," and he held his hand out, palm up, as if it were slightly weighted with the human heart . . . "[and] he don't know no more about it than you or me."
                                    —Flannery O'Connor, "The Life You Save
                                                  May Be Your Own"

Christmas Eve 2001, Fargo. The view from my parents' living room was serene. Tree boughs speckled white split like dendrites onto the gray sky. Inside the house, piles of snowshoes were stowed in the foyer. Our guests were sitting in animated conversation, men and women separately, as was always the case at my parents' holiday parties in North Dakota, where my parents had moved for my father's genetics professorship before I entered medical school. In the kitchen, Vinny Shah, a cardiac surgeon and family friend, found me. He had just been called to operate on a patient with endocarditis, an infection of the mitral valve, which separates the left atrium from the left ventricle.

Acute infectious endocarditis is one of the deadliest diseases. The risk of death among some patients starts at around 20 percent and gallops in 1 or 2 percent increments per hour. Sir William Osler, the famed Canadian physician who founded the first residency program in the United States, at Johns Hopkins, noted that "few diseases present greater difficulty" and that "in fully one-half the diagnosis is made post-mortem." Setting down his plate, Shah asked me, a first-year fellow, if I wanted to come along and watch. But there was no time to lose.

Outside, my breath smoked vaporously in the frigid air. We slipped and slid our way on salted roads to the hospital. The facility was a collection of solitary buildings—flat, rectangular—sitting in a bleak white landscape. The lot had been plowed, but the few cars that were parked were blanketed with snow, their wipers pointing up, as if in surrender. Our feet crunched on the frozen ground as we made our way to the entrance. In front of the gift shop, closed for the holiday, a young man in scrubs and a snow jacket, a surgical tech, was smoking a cigarette. He quietly followed us in.

The operating room on the second floor had a strangely ad hoc quality, as if no one had planned on being there that night. Instruments were scattered about and tables were askew. The air smelled vaguely industrial, like a photographic darkroom. The staff was moving purposefully, almost noiselessly. They looked like the sorts of people you might find working at Walmart on a Saturday night. A scrub nurse was adding and subtracting scalpels and spatulas on a sterile drape. An anesthesiologist was fiddling with stopcocks and syringes. A surgical assistant was getting ready to insert a catheter. The odd one of the bunch was the beefy perfusionist sitting on a stool by the heart-lung machine. He was reading a magazine.

The patient was lying on a bench in the corner of the room, getting prepped. He seemed blank, listless, having had night sweats and debilitating fatigue for weeks. Up close I noticed he had long gray hair, like a hippie, and pools of black ink for eyes.

His ribs poked out of his bony chest like spokes on a wheel. Congested veins rippled on his wasted temples. Like that of many elderly patients, his skin was imprinted with purplish blotches where IVs had leaked blood. His echocardiogram showed vegetations—cheesy specks of infectious material—on both mitral leaflets, flapping around like flags in the wind. The bottom leaflet had been partially eaten away, leaving a gap through which blood was leaking back into the left atrium and farther back into the lungs, filling the air sacs with fluid, slowly drowning him. This was the reason he could not catch his breath.

Shah and I introduced ourselves. The man turned to us slowly, not really looking at us. "Am I ready for the glue factory?" he said.

In the dressing room, I pulled off my slacks and folded and snapped them under the bright lights. I hung up my clothes in a locker and put on green scrubs, like the kind I'd worn in anatomy lab in St. Louis six years prior. At the metal washbasin, Shah and I scrubbed our hands and arms to the elbow with brown iodinated soap. He spoke with a slightly oblique tone that seemed to intimate that there was more to what he was saying, even when he was saying something pretty obvious. "This man is sick," he intoned gravely, kicking an aluminum panel to turn off the faucet. "If we don't operate tonight, he will die." I said nothing. It was my first heart surgery, and I wasn't sure what to say or do. Should I ask questions and try to learn something? Or keep my mouth shut and stay out of the way?

Back in the OR, we donned sterile gowns and gloves and blue masks. Everything in the room was gray, beige, or blue, save for the wildly colored surgical caps. Shah put on tiny binoculars, like a jeweler's spectacles. He was a handsome man, tall and lanky, with coiffed jet-black hair, like a Bollywood actor's, only partially covered by his paisley beret. "Stand here, next to me, but don't touch anything," he said. He grabbed the sterile plastic cover on the ceiling lamp and adjusted the light just so.

By now the patient was anesthetized and intubated, looking like just another cadaver. A mess of tubes and wires slithered menacingly across the table toward him. The operation was ready to begin.

With a scalpel, Shah cut through the skin over the breastbone. A necklace of dark red beads quickly appeared. With a buzz saw that looked like an ironing press, Shah made a linear cut along the entire length of the sternum. His assistant quickly poked at tiny bleeding vessels with a cautery, liberating tiny puffs of proteinaceous smoke. Using a stainless-steel retractor, they separated the two sides of the sternum, and the pink-and-yellow chest cavity came into view. Holding forceps and a scalpel, Shah cut open the silvery pericardium. The heart was dancing wildly, an incredible sight. I thought back to those dog days of summer in St. Louis, but what I beheld was so different from the dry brown heart of my nameless cadaver. This one was pink, like uncooked chicken; for a moment, it seemed to be the only thing in the room that was moving. Plastic catheters were quickly stitched into the right atrium and the aorta. They would be used to create a circuit for the heart-lung machine that was going to keep our patient alive.

The machine itself was a beige box, about the size of a small refrigerator, with a dizzying array of dials and tubes. It had already been primed with saline to purge it of air. Shah connected the machine via hoses to the catheters in the chest and told the perfusionist to turn it on. When he did, incredibly the heart began to shrink as blood, life's fluid, was diverted into the plastic-and-metal apparatus. The heart nevertheless continued to beat, though weakly and more slowly. Much of my life I'd lived with the fear that the heart could stop at any moment and one's life would be extinguished. And here it was, shrinking like a balloon with a small leak. It sent shivers through me. Never had the boundary between life and death seemed so thin.

With a metal clamp, Shah compressed the aorta, cutting off blood flow from the heart, thus isolating it. Then he injected ice-cold potassium solution into the main cardiac vein. Concentrated potassium is used to stop the heart in executions, and sure enough the patient's EKG quickly flatlined. Shah poured iced saline directly on the heart to cool it further. Then, with the heart quarantined and the patient's circulation and oxygenation being controlled by the heart-lung machine, he began to cut into the diseased organ.

•

Many (mostly American) breakthroughs allowed that Christmas Eve surgery to take place, but perhaps none was bigger than the heart-lung machine. It has been described by the physician and author James Le Fanu as "among the boldest and most successful feats of man's mind." The machine was conceived by John Gibbon, a Philadelphia surgeon, in 1930, but it took almost twenty-five years to develop. One reason for the delay was the economic downturn during the Great Depression, and then there was World War II. But progress was also retarded by cultural fallacies. Though an artificial kidney was developed with relatively little fanfare, the heart occupied a special place in the popular imagination. How could a man-made machine replace the organ that houses the soul?

Without such a machine, cardiac surgeons were hamstrung. Once the heart is stopped to cut it open, a timer starts to tick. Deprived of oxygen-rich blood from the heart, the brain and vital organs will get irreversibly damaged within three to five minutes. However, most congenital heart malformations require at least ten minutes of circulatory stoppage to repair, too long to avoid brain injury. So, most surgeons believed such operations could never be performed, at least not until a machine was built to take over heart and lung function for those crucial minutes.

One surgeon who believed there was an alternative was C. Walton Lillehei, considered by many the most innovative surgeon of the twentieth century. Born and raised in Minneapolis, Lillehei grew up an inveterate tinkerer. As a teenager, when his parents refused to buy him a motorcycle, he built one out of spare parts. He brought that engineering mentality to his surgical research. His small research lab in the attic of Millard Hall at the University of Minnesota was nothing more than two operating tables, a sink, and a few oxygen tanks. But it was there, following his chief Owen Wangensteen's edict to transform the department into a center of surgical invention, that Lillehei developed perhaps the most bizarre idea in the history of surgery: controlled cross-circulation.

Lillehei's ideas were inspired by the circulation of blood between mother and fetus in mammals. Because the fetus is bathed in amniotic fluid, it cannot obtain oxygen by taking breaths. Its blood must be shunted into the mother, where it is oxygenated and cleaned of waste before returning to the fetus. Why, Lillehei reasoned, couldn't the same scheme be employed in heart surgery? An animal (a "donor") could be used to clean and oxygenate blood from another animal (the "recipient"), returning the blood to the recipient to nourish it while the recipient's heart was stopped and isolated from the circulation. It seemed so simple, circumventing the need for a machine. In Lillehei's early experiments, the circulatory systems of two anesthetized dogs were connected through a beer hose to a milk pump between them that pushed equal amounts of blood in opposite directions without introducing air bubbles. With the recipient dog's chest splayed open, the inlet and outlet of its heart were clamped off, its lungs collapsed, and its blue venous blood propelled by the milk pump into the donor dog. Red, oxygenated blood was returned from the donor to the recipient through an artery in the recipient's chest. In this way, the donor served as the recipient's heart and lungs while the recipient's heart was stopped and drained of blood.

At first, Lillehei and his team made mistakes in the complex hookup of the circuit, and the dogs, which they'd picked up from the pound, suffered brain damage. But after a few attempts, they were able to carry out their experiments successfully, with both recipient and donor dogs waking up unscathed.

After the experiments, the dogs were euthanized and their organs examined under a microscope. There was no evidence that cross-circulation caused damage to either animal. The recipient was supplied with enough blood and oxygen to maintain basic function, and the donor's ability to circulate its own blood wasn't compromised either. A few months later, Lillehei tested his method on trained dogs, including the purebred golden retrievers of a cardiologist colleague. Even after thirty minutes of cross-circulation, the dogs were still able to follow commands and do their usual tricks.

In 1954, after years of experiments on some two hundred dogs, Lillehei and his team were eager to try their method on humans. They were interested in correcting congenital heart defects. At the time, fifty thousand or so American babies were born every year with such anomalies. (Even today, a baby is born with a heart defect in the United States every fifteen minutes.) Most defects are coin-sized holes in the wall between the atria or the ventricles, allowing mixing of oxygen-rich and oxygen-poor blood. These holes can result in stunted growth, oxygen deprivation, fainting, even sudden death. "Congenitals" were a fixture on hospital wards in the 1950s, often seen sitting on the edges of their beds, leaning forward to catch their breath, legs distended like tree trunks, seeping pale yellow fluid (the result of congestive heart failure) through their skin and into puddles on the tile floor. They frequently had facial deformities because heart defects often coexist with anomalies like Down syndrome. They suffered crippling infections, too; half died before the age of twenty. In short, they were cardiac cripples, their existence doomed, their prognosis worse than many childhood cancers. A leading surgeon asserted that it should be possible to fix some of the heart anomalies "as a plumber changes pipes around," but such surgery was prohibitively long.

Though the need was great, Lillehei's proposal to use one human as living circuitry for another was shocking, to some even immoral: the first operation in human history that had the potential to kill two people. The idea of anesthetizing a normal human being in the operating room to provide life support to another while the other's heart was stopped, sliced open, and repaired was unacceptable to most doctors, a violation of their most fundamental oath. However, with no artificial heart-lung machine available, and despite the fervid opposition of his colleagues, Lillehei forged ahead.

Lillehei had one attribute that set him apart from most other doctors: he was a cancer survivor. In his final year of residency, he had been diagnosed with a usually fatal lymphosarcoma of the neck. No less than Wangensteen, his department chief, operated on him in a ten-and-a-half-hour surgery. Lillehei's biopsy results had actually come in several months prior, but Wangensteen had waited until a few days before Lillehei graduated to tell him so the young surgeon would finish his residency. In the operation, Wangensteen and his team excised the tumor, lymph nodes, and much of the surrounding soft tissue of Lillehei's chest and neck. Exploratory surgery a few months later showed no trace of cancer.

With such a close brush with mortality, Lillehei seemed to have a better acquaintance with death than most surgeons, rendering him less fearful of it. He had been given a 25 percent chance of surviving five years, so for much of his early career he was running along the edge of a precipice, waiting for the inevitable slip that would send him into the abyss. His tenuous hold on his own life conferred courage, perhaps even a kind of foolhardiness. He was going to spend whatever time remained for him tackling the conundrum of open-heart surgery. He was willing to try new things, experimental procedures with low chances of success, despite the up-front costs. For his part, Wangensteen gave Lillehei the time and resources to perform his innovative work. He was protective over him like a father over a vulnerable child. He was also convinced that Lillehei had the best chance of any of his protégés to be awarded a Nobel Prize.

There was another alternative to the heart-lung machine

besides cross-circulation, at least for simple heart surgeries: cooling the body down to freezing temperatures to slow the metabolism and thus reduce the need for oxygen. A ten-degree drop in temperature halves the rate of most chemical reactions, including cellular processes, which is why people have been known to survive submerged in a frozen lake for up to forty minutes. The first use of surgical hypothermia was presented by Wilfred Bigelow, a Canadian surgeon, at a conference in Denver in 1950. Bigelow anesthetized laboratory dogs, cooled them in an ice bath, opened their chests, clamped off their hearts to stop blood flow, and then de-clamped, stitched, warmed, and woke them up with no permanent brain damage. He later found that monkeys were even better than dogs at tolerating hypothermia. At sixty-eight degrees Fahrenheit, they could have their circulation stopped for almost twenty minutes with no damage to their brain function.*

The first successful human demonstration of Bigelow's "frozen lake" strategy took place on September 2, 1952—more than half a century after Ludwig Rehn's first myocardial stitch—when Dr. John Lewis, a slightly senior colleague of Lillehei's at the University of Minnesota, used hypothermia to fix an "atrial septal defect," a hole in the wall between the left and right atria, in a five-year-old girl named Jacqueline Johnson. Though the girl's heart was enlarged, she herself was frail and underweight. She had been sick for most of her life with recurrent pneumonia, and doctors had written her off as having only a few years to live. Faced with such a grim prognosis, her parents gave Lewis and his team the go-ahead to operate.

Using a rubber blanket that circulated a cold alcohol solution, Lewis cooled Jacqueline's core body temperature over many hours, the thermometer reading steadily dropping from normal, around 98.6 degrees Fahrenheit, down to 79 degrees.

*Hypothermia was also tried as a treatment for metastatic cancer, leukemia, schizophrenia, and drug addiction, with discouraging results.

He quickly pinched off her major veins and arteries with tourniquets so that no blood could get into or out of her heart, achieving an almost bloodless organ. At this point, no blood was circulating in her frozen body. Then, with a scalpel, he cut through the wall of her right atrium, being careful to avoid the coronary arteries and essential electrical structures. It took about three minutes for him to find the dime-sized hole. Within two minutes, he had sewn it shut. To test the repair's integrity, he injected the heart with salt water to make sure there was no leak. When it looked as if the repair was intact, he released the clamps on the major blood vessels. The heart began to beat sluggishly. With his hands in the open chest, Lewis massaged it, willing it by hand to do its job, and within a few minutes the heart began to speed up. After a few minutes, Lewis warmed up the little girl in room-temperature water, filling a trough that had been purchased from Sears, Roebuck. Though there were a few small bumps in her postoperative course, Jacqueline did well. Eleven days after the operation, she went home. By the end of the month, she was just another girl at school.

The acclaim for Wangensteen and his department was widespread. "'Deep Freeze' Heart Girl Making Rapid Recovery," announced a headline in *The New York Times*. *The Minneapolis Tribune* gushed that the operation "seems to give surgeons a method, long sought, of putting the knife to the live human heart in plain sight." Though many who opposed animal experimentation were aghast, a newspaper editorialist, referring to the number of dogs that had been sacrificed in developing the technique, wrote that "one child at the price of fourteen dogs is a remarkable bargain."

Still, hypothermia wasn't the blanket answer for all congenital heart defects. It afforded surgeons only a fraction of the time they needed because it protected the non-perfused brain for only a relatively short period. While five minutes was sufficient time to repair a simple lesion like an atrial septal defect (ASD), more complex defects, such as ventricular septal defects

(VSDs), the most common type of congenital heart abnormality, in which holes in the wall separating the two ventricles allow blood to flow abnormally, required more time, at least ten minutes. And so, these patients continued to be labeled "inoperable."

Lillehei proposed using cross-circulation on these children. He appealed to Wangensteen, expecting his full support, but the chief refused to grant him permission. The technique was too new, Wangensteen said, too risky to use on a frail child, and he correctly predicted the furor that would erupt if a child not facing imminent death—or his donor parent—succumbed on the operating table. Lillehei pushed on, presenting Wangensteen with published reports showing poor outcomes of experimental VSD repairs using the hypothermia method, but Wangensteen was unmoved. He gave permission to Lewis, Lillehei's rival, to perform the first VSD repair using hypothermia. Only after Lewis quickly failed in his first two attempts, resulting in two deaths, did Wangensteen relent and give Lillehei the opportunity he had been waiting for.

Lillehei's first patient was a thirteen-month-old boy with a VSD. Gregory Glidden, as he was named, lived with his parents and eight siblings in the north woods of Minnesota about a hundred miles from Minneapolis. His father, Lyman, a mine worker, and his mother, Frances, were tragically familiar with congenital heart disease. Gregory's older sister had also been born with a VSD and had died unexpectedly in her sleep three and a half years earlier. (Frances found her dead in bed one morning.) Like his sister, Gregory had spent most of his young life in the hospital. His first words and first steps were spoken and taken on a lonely patient ward. In December 1953, Gregory's pediatrician sent an urgent referral to the University of Minnesota. The little boy was having frequent fevers and could not easily draw breath. He weighed just eleven pounds, no more than his stuffed animals. His heart was enlarging, too, at an alarming rate; it was more than double the normal size, a sign of impending circulatory failure.

Cardiologists in Minneapolis admitted Gregory to the Variety Club Heart Hospital at the University of Minnesota. After performing tests to confirm the presence of the VSD, they arranged for a consultation with Lillehei. They had heard about the innovative research he was doing in the attic of Millard Hall. Perhaps this maverick would be the one to finally fix the dreaded VSD and prevent another baby's death. After meeting Gregory, Lillehei proposed an operation in which he would fix the boy's VSD using cross-circulation, with Lyman Glidden, who had his son's blood type, serving as the donor. Lillehei made it clear to the Gliddens that he had used cross-circulation only on dogs, but he told them that if a child of his needed open-heart surgery, he would not hesitate to use the technique. Desperate, the Gliddens gave the go-ahead. The consent form they signed in March 1954 was a single sentence: "I, the undersigned, hereby grant permission for an operation or any procedure the University staff deems necessary upon my son."

Today, patient autonomy and shared decision making are mantras in the hospital, ethical imperatives that supersede all others, including beneficence. But the situation was very different in the 1950s, when doctors were more apt to act without what we would consider informed consent. Medical paternalism was rampant, but it would be a mistake to think of Lillehei as authoritarian. By all accounts, he was an unusually compassionate physician, having been a patient himself. As a patient, he knew the vulnerability that comes with illness. He knew on a visceral level how patients look to their doctors for guidance and protection. But as a surgeon, he also understood that his young patients had no chance for a normal life and that there were no other procedures available to help them. Desperate parents did not want to hear that there were no options. They wanted a doctor to do—try—something.

As a father, I can only imagine the Gliddens' agony. I can see them racing across the flat Minnesota landscape that winter, sick child in tow, the white dashes on the straight road extending like a zipper to the horizon. They were still mourning their daughter and were desperate to avoid another young death in their family. Their hearts were full of fear—the worst kind, of love about to be snatched away—but courage, too: the courage to go first, to offer up their little boy for a chance, however small, at a normal life, and perhaps for the sake of science as well.

Lillehei's experiments are a painful reminder that innovation and expertise in medicine are earned on patients, and unfortunately there is always a learning curve. How to protect patients while doctors learn is a conundrum still faced in all areas of medicine. For example, in the early 1990s, a hospital in Bristol, England, introduced an innovative operation to correct a congenital heart abnormality in babies called transposition of the great arteries. Before this, newborns with this condition were treated with a palliative procedure that had poor long-term outcomes. Children at the hospital ultimately benefited from the innovation, but a heavy price was paid. The death rate for babies in the first few years after doctors started doing the operation was many times higher than with the palliative procedure. Commenting on the poor outcomes, a pediatric surgeon wrote that it was understood "there would initially be a period of disappointing results."

Observers were aghast, however, calling for a moratorium on the procedure. They argued that surgeons with children's lives in their hands should not take on more than they could handle. How then, surgeons responded, do we innovate? For a new technology, there is no opportunity for rehearsal. For an innovation to benefit patients, there has to be a first time.

There seems to have been no hand-wringing on Lillehei's part, no soul-searching about how to protect babies and children while he learned on them. The kids, Lillehei knew, were doomed anyway, justifying the risks. But he underestimated the backlash. Even the hospital was against him. In the afternoon before the operation, Cecil Watson, chief of medicine, and Irvine McQuarrie, chief of pediatrics, wrote a letter to the head of the

medical center demanding that the surgery be aborted. There
was too much to lose, not just a little boy and his healthy father,
but also the hospital's reputation as the first heart institute in
the country. It had taken years to earn this title, and they were
not about to let a young upstart surgeon slow their momen-
tum. However, the director, Ray Amberg, refused to intervene.
He would not get involved in medical matters, he said, giving
Lillehei a de facto green light to proceed.

The operating theater that late-March morning was packed
with onlookers. Lying on a table was Gregory, still clutching
his teddy bear. An injection of sodium pentothal rendered him
unconscious. After a breathing tube was inserted, Lillehei
worked quickly. He made an incision across the tiny chest. He
split the fragile breastbone. Once the walnut-sized heart came
into view, he called for Lyman, the father, who was wheeled in
by stretcher and placed three feet from his son. He, too, was
quickly sedated, but only lightly, lest the medicine in his bloodstream poison the boy. Watching them, Lillehei knew that if
his technique did not work, father and son could very well be
buried this way.

Lillehei inserted plastic catheters into Gregory, while his
assistants inserted separate catheters into Lyman. The boy was
then connected to his father, vein to vein, artery to artery, via
a beer hose passing through a Sigmamotor milk pump. Lillehei's team had to be careful: too little blood through the pump
would result in oxygen deprivation to Gregory's organs; too
much could cause brain swelling and tissue edema. After the
pump was turned on (and confirmed not to leak), Lillehei tied
off all inlets and outlets to Gregory's heart, isolating it from
the circulation. At that point, Lyman Glidden's heart and lungs
were keeping both father and son alive—just as a mother's
would for her developing child.

For thirteen and a half minutes, well past the time that hypothermia could afford, Lillehei operated on the bluish plum
in Gregory's chest. He cut through the outer wall of the heart.

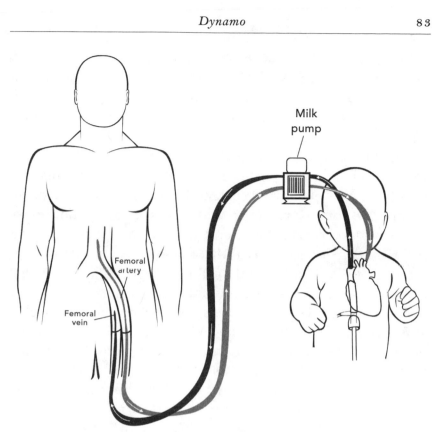

Circuit used for Lillehei's first cross-circulation operation (Created by Liam Eisenberg, Koyo Designs)

With a relatively bloodless environment, visibility was good. He quickly found the VSD. It could have been any number of morphologies—a single hole, a tear, a flapping membrane involving the valves, even a Swiss cheese pattern—but fortunately for Lillehei (and his patient) that day, it was an isolated dime-sized hole high up in the ventricular septum. He sewed it closed with a dozen silk stitches.

After he was done, Lillehei's assistants released the tourniquet around Gregory's venae cavae, allowing blood to return to his heart. Almost immediately—and to everyone's surprise, none more than Lillehei's—it started to beat vigorously. The milk pump was turned off, father and son were quickly separated, and their wounds closed. Lillehei and a relieved assistant reached across the boy and shook hands. The patients were sent to separate recovery rooms. A few hours later, Lillehei informed Frances that her husband and son were awake and intact.

For the first few days, Gregory's postoperative course was smooth. Though groggy from painkillers, he drank milk and took some bites of poached egg and Cream of Wheat. But pneumonia, "the old man's best friend," as Osler once said, set in. Gregory's lips turned blue, and his breaths quickened. His trachea was suctioned constantly of bloody mucus. Though he received the most powerful antibiotics, his condition worsened. Near the end, anesthesiologists were squeezing oxygen from a bag directly into his lungs. On the morning of April 6, 1954, eleven days after the historic operation, Gregory Glidden's heart finally stopped. An autopsy showed the cause of death was a chest infection. His VSD remained closed.

Despite the setback, Lillehei decided to perform another VSD repair two weeks later, this time on a four-year-old girl named Pamela Schmidt who had lived in an oxygen tent for almost a year. She was battling pneumonia when Lillehei first met her, so he had to wait for penicillin to do its job. During the four-and-a-half-hour operation, Schmidt's heart was separated from her circulatory system for nearly fourteen minutes. But this time, Lillehei's patient survived the surgery. Her father, the donor, also recovered uneventfully.

On April 30, 1954, Lillehei held a press conference in Minneapolis to describe his cross-circulation technique. He showed slides describing the pathology of the VSD and talked about his failed first attempt on Gregory Glidden. Then he introduced Pamela, a brown-haired beauty, who was pushed across the stage in a wheelchair. The reporters were thrilled, and Lillehei's operation became a worldwide sensation. *Time* called it "daring." *The New York Times* deemed it "impossible." London's *Daily Mirror* proclaimed it "as extravagant and fantastic as any ever written in a shilling science thriller." Pamela became a national celebrity, too, appearing on television and in a six-page photo spread in *Cosmopolitan*. The American Heart Association dubbed her "the Queen of Hearts."

But Lillehei, no stranger to tragedy, did not forget about Lyman and Frances Glidden. A few weeks earlier, unable to afford a headstone, they had buried Gregory in an unmarked grave next to his sister. On May 4, Lillehei sent them a letter. "It is still a source of bitter disappointment to me that we were not able to bring Gregory through the post-operative period after the operation had seemingly gone so well," he wrote. "I do wish to tell you again that had it not been for the encouragement gained from Gregory's operation, we would not have had the courage to go ahead . . . I feel greatly indebted to both of you." Perhaps the world did, too.

During the spring and summer of 1954, Lillehei was the only person on the planet performing advanced open-heart surgery. His surgical suite, according to a visitor, the British cardiac surgeon Donald Ross, "was like a circus. There was a large gallery in the operating room with about fifty people. People were rushing in and rushing out . . . The operating room was chaos, with pipes and tubes everywhere." But his patients did well.

However, that autumn, Lillehei went through a spell of extraordinarily bad luck. Six out of seven cross-circulation cases ended in death. In one operation in October, a donor mother suffered severe brain damage after an anesthesiologist inadvertently injected air into her IV line. Tense colleagues whispered that Lillehei was a "murderer"; no one could stomach seeing little babies die. In response, Lillehei reportedly said, "You don't venture into a wilderness expecting to find a paved road."

Lillehei continued to use cross-circulation for several more years, correcting increasingly complex congenital defects. He searched for voluntary donors in unusual places, including the state penitentiary. When white inmates refused to serve as a donor for a black man, Lillehei decided to use a dog's lung to oxygenate that patient's blood. The man quickly succumbed on the operating table.

Despite isolated successes, cross-circulation fell out of favor. "We are still convinced that it is preferable to perform operations . . . by some procedure which does not involve another healthy person," John Gibbon, a professor of surgery in Philadelphia who had been working on a heart-lung machine for two decades, declared. Lillehei himself had abandoned the technique by the late 1950s. In the end, he performed forty-five operations with it, with twenty-eight long-term survivors, a mortality rate of 40 percent, which was still better than the natural prognosis of uncorrected congenital defects. In the end, history has judged his work to be a success.

By the mid-1950s, a prototype of a heart-lung machine had been built and was ready to be used on humans. "It would provide surgeons with a dry field for operation, permitting for the first time the fullest use of their most valuable assets—their hands and eyes," the renowned surgeon Claude Beck said at Case Western Reserve University in Cleveland in 1951. The machine was a massive technological leap, but it required an equally large conceptual jump: that blood could be circulated and oxygenated by a machine; that in the end there was nothing fundamentally special about the human heart.

5

Pump

We are in large part recompensed for the long and difficult hours by seeing the most miraculous change in the
children and in witnessing the joy and relief of the parents when they see their children running about happily
and without effort like other children.
—Lord Brock, cardiac surgeon,
Guy's Hospital, London

The scale of heart disease in the 1950s was like that of AIDS
in the 1980s: a disease that dominated American medicine both
clinically and politically. More than 600,000 Americans were
dying of heart disease every year. In 1945, the budget for
medical research at the National Institutes of Health was
$180,000. Five years later, it was $46 million. A large portion
went to cardiac research, in part because of political advocacy
by the American Heart Association and other lobbies. In 1950,
President Harry Truman, in a warning about heart disease
starkly similar to the one he delivered about the Iron Curtain
spreading across Europe, said that "measures to cope with this
threat are of immediate concern to every one of us."

It still amazes me that so many advances in heart treatment

occurred in the decade just after my grandfather died, and so many of them in Minnesota, too, only a few hours' drive from the hospital in Fargo where I stood with Dr. Shah in the operating room that Christmas morning. Our patient's open chest was framed by sterile towels, like blue curtains stained with punch. Shah's red-streaked fingers moved surely, precisely, as if each digit were following a programmed script. We were about fifteen minutes in, the heart quivering in fibrillation, when he applied blade to muscle and sliced open the left atrium. Tears of blood streamed from the slit. He reached into the heart and pulled up on the patient's infected mitral valve with sutures, urging me to come in closer for a better view. The infected growths on the leaflets were small and white, like a baby's teeth, and seemingly just as innocuous. It was hard to believe they had almost killed the man.

One thing I'll never forget is how relaxed Shah appeared. He talked about the town, the weather, his friendship with my parents, residency training, even his belief that elderly patients with less time left to them have a greater will to live than younger patients. He took every opportunity to explain what he was doing, perhaps sensitive about shortchanging my investment of time on a major holiday. There was none of the slow panic I expected after the patient's chest was opened. At one point, Shah inserted his finger into a bleeding hole and turned to me like a man waiting for a train. "We want to use a tissue, not metal, valve because at his age we don't want him on long-term blood thinners." I nodded nervously. I couldn't believe that even at that tense moment, Shah was trying to teach me something. Of course, he could afford to take his time because the heart-lung machine was keeping our patient alive. Without it, the atmosphere in the OR would have been very different.

•

The person who contributed most to the invention of the heart-lung machine was a similarly generous, if ambivalent, soul. Toward the end of his first year at Jefferson Medical College in

Philadelphia, John Heysham Gibbon Jr. considered quitting medicine to become a writer, a passion he'd nurtured since his college years at Princeton. His father, a pragmatist, advised him to obtain his medical degree, telling him (in advice that sounds very familiar) that he would not "write worse for having it." So Gibbon persevered and received his MD three years later, in 1927.

During his internship at Boston City Hospital, he began to toy with the idea of "extracorporeal circulation." One night, his research mentor, Edward Churchill, had him monitor a dying young woman who had developed a massive lung clot after a routine gallbladder operation. Churchill knew that incising the blood-filled pulmonary arteries to evacuate the clot, an operation called a pulmonary embolectomy, would almost certainly result in fatal bleeding. But isolating the heart to prevent

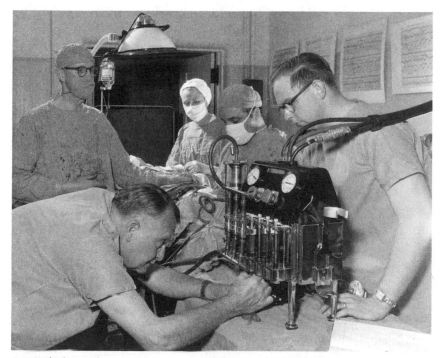

An early heart-lung machine, circa 1954 (Courtesy of Walter P. Reuther Library, Archives of Labor and Urban Affairs, Wayne State University)

exsanguination was not an option; without oxygen delivery, the brain would get irreversibly damaged within minutes. The pulmonary embolectomy operation was invented in 1908 by Friedrich Trendelenburg, a German surgeon, but none of his patients survived. "Twelve times we have done it at the clinic," he lamented in 1912, "my assistants oftener than myself, and not once with success." Noting this horrible mortality, Trendelenburg's contemporary, the Swedish surgeon Gunnar Nyström, said, "Our rule is not to operate until the patient, as far as is humanly possible to judge, no longer has any chance of returning to life."*

So Churchill, stuck in a surgical catch-22, vacillated. Perhaps the clot would dissolve on its own or crumble and migrate down smaller arterial byways. Perhaps other areas of the lung would increase ventilation to compensate. He instructed Gibbon to notify him when the patient's condition became so tenuous, so near death, that a Hail Mary operation would be justified. Early the following morning, as the patient's blood pressure dived and she became unresponsive, Gibbon called his chief. The woman was rushed to the operating room but died on the table.†

Though Gibbon was a stoic researcher more comfortable around pipettes than people, he wept over that young woman. But in her death, he had a eureka moment. "During that long night," he said in 1970, "helplessly watching the patient struggle for life as her blood became darker and her veins more distended, the idea naturally occurred to me that if it were possible to remove continuously some of the blue blood from the patient's swollen veins, put oxygen into that blood and allow

*Edward Churchill himself said in 1934, "Although our enthusiasm is somewhat dampened by a series of ten failures, we shall continue to recommend the Trendelenburg operation under favorable circumstances."
†The first successful pulmonary embolectomy in America took place at the Peter Bent Brigham Hospital in Boston on January 14, 1958, well after the invention of the heart-lung machine.

carbon dioxide to escape from it, and then to inject continuously the now-red blood back into the patient's arteries, we might have saved her life. We would have bypassed the obstructing embolus and performed part of the work of the patient's heart and lungs outside the body."

Gibbon and his research assistant (and wife), Mary Hopkinson, essentially devoted the rest of their professional lives to this goal. His mentors discouraged him, believing that his outsized ambition would be better spent on a less risky project. Churchill himself took a "dim" view of the proposed work. In the medical academy, then as now, huge outlays of time and money for big ideas were frowned upon. In a publish-or-perish world, you had to get your name in the top journals with regularity. Gibbon's mentors advised him to pursue iterative problems, problems whose solutions might tweak the existing paradigm but would not try to supplant it.

However, Gibbon had a stick-to-itiveness that was unusual, even for a medical scientist, and so he applied himself and forged on. The result was a thirty-year academic career devoted to one big idea. But it changed medicine forever.

What Gibbon faced was an engineering problem: how to drain blood from the body, oxygenate it in a machine of metal and plastic without forming clots,* and then pump it back into the body without air bubbles to nourish the vital organs. To solve this problem, he needed animals. He and Mary performed their early experiments on stray cats they plucked with tuna fish bait and a gunnysack from the streets of Boston. They went to the lab early in the morning because the preparations for their experiments took several hours. They would anesthetize a cat, perform a tracheotomy, and connect the animal to an artificial

---

*The clotting problem was solved with the use of heparin, a blood-thinning protein discovered by Jay McLean, a medical student at Johns Hopkins, in the brains of salamanders. (The substance was initially called cephalin.) In the 1920s, animal experiments confirmed that heparin was an effective anticoagulant.

respirator. By mid-afternoon, they were ready to start the main demonstration: sucking blood out of the animal, circulating it through a machine while the heart was stopped, and then pumping it back into the animal to keep it alive. After much trial and error, they settled on the following scheme: isolate the cat's heart by tying off the major veins and arteries; withdraw blood from a vein in the head at a rate of about half a soda can per minute; pass it in a thin stream down a rotating metal cylinder in an atmosphere of almost pure oxygen, which allowed the blood to pick up oxygen and give up carbon dioxide through diffusion; and finally collect the blood at the bottom of the cylinder, warm it, and return it to an artery in the animal's leg via an air pump, which Gibbon purchased for a few dollars at a secondhand shop near the hospital. Mary later said, "We would keep the clamp completely occluding the pulmonary artery for as long as we thought the cat could stand it, or nothing went wrong with the apparatus, but things that were apt to go wrong were infinite."

Their machine was, as Gibbon described it, an assemblage of "metal, glass, electric motors, water baths, electrical switches, electromagnets, etc. . . . [that] looked for all the world like some ridiculous Rube Goldberg apparatus." It went through numerous refinements through the 1930s, eventually growing to the size of a grand piano. But inelegant as it was, it worked. By the end of the decade, Gibbon could keep cats and dogs alive for several hours and, most important, was able to wean the animals off the machine to resume their own heart and lung function. In 1939, Gibbon published his findings in a paper titled "The Maintenance of Life During Experimental Occlusion of the Pulmonary Artery Followed by Survival." He later wrote, "I will never forget the day when we were able to screw the clamp down all the way, completely occluding the pulmonary artery, with the extracorporeal blood circuit in operation and with no change in the animal's blood pressure. My wife and I threw our arms around each other and danced around the laboratory laughing and shouting hooray." He added, "Although it gives great satisfaction to me and others to know that the [heart] operations are being performed daily now all over the world, nothing in my life has duplicated the ecstasy and joy of that dance with Mary around the laboratory of the old Bulfinch building in the Massachusetts General Hospital."

Humans are a lot bigger than cats, however; we have roughly eight times the blood volume of a feline. So Gibbon began to think of ways to adapt his machine for human use. His research was interrupted when he was called to serve as a trauma surgeon in the Pacific theater from 1941 to 1945. After the war, when Gibbon returned to his project, major problems still needed to be solved. Blood cells were getting chewed up in the pump. Particles of protein, fibrin, fat, and gas were injuring vital organs. And of course, a larger machine was required to handle the greater blood volume in humans—no longer a soda can but a milk gallon. To help him solve these problems, Gibbon turned to the IBM Corporation, whose chairman, Thomas Watson, was the father-in-law of one of his students. With the aid of IBM's engineers, Gibbon refined his machine: adding filters to catch clots, increasing the size of the oxygenator, and incorporating special roller pumps. The postwar years were ripe for such research. Large-scale public-private projects were being launched in computing, nuclear technology, and space exploration. Gibbon's team took advantage of this political environment to essentially compress three billion years of evolution into two decades of intense human endeavor. By the early 1950s, the mortality rate in his animal experiments had decreased from 80 percent to 12 percent, and Gibbon believed the time had come to try his machine on a human being.

Gibbon wasn't the only scientist working on a heart-lung machine. Between 1950 and 1955, five medical centers were engaged in the pursuit, each with a different design. At the University of Toronto, William Mustard developed a machine that used isolated rhesus monkey lungs to oxygenate the blood.

At Wayne State University in Detroit, Forest Dodrill and engineers from General Motors built a heart pump that looked very much like the engine in a Cadillac. At the Mayo Clinic, John Kirklin and his colleagues constructed a heart-lung machine based on Gibbon's design that used a vertical oxygenator and roller pumps (it was eventually called the Mayo-Gibbon oxygenator). At the University of Minnesota, Clarence Dennis, a colleague of Lillehei's, developed his own machine based on drawings that Gibbon had shared with him on a visit to Gibbon's lab. Dennis would be the first to try the heart-lung machine on a human, six-year-old Patty Anderson, who would die on the operating table. His next attempt also failed when assistants let the reservoir run dry, pumping air into the patient's arteries, killing her instantly. From 1951 to 1953, eighteen patients were reported to have undergone open-heart surgery with heart-lung machine support. Seventeen died.

It is only fitting that Gibbon, who conceived of the heart-lung machine and worked on it longer than anyone else, was the first, and not Dennis, to use it successfully on a person. Gibbon's first attempt, after decades of animal experiments, proved tragic when the fifteen-month-old baby bled to death as he frantically searched for an atrial septal defect she did not have. (She had been misdiagnosed.) On March 27, 1953, he tried again, this time on Cecelia Bavolek, an eighteen-year-old freshman at Wilkes College in Pennsylvania. She had been hospitalized with heart failure three times in the previous six months. The surgery to repair her ASD took more than five hours. Managed by six assistants and weighing more than a ton, Gibbon's machine took over the patient's circulation for approximately thirty minutes while he sewed the half-dollar-sized hole closed with cotton sutures. The operation had an unexpected complication: the machine clogged because it ran out of blood thinner and had to be operated manually. When Gibbon took Bavolek off the machine, he had low expectations. But her young heart restarted almost immediately. One hour after he closed up her

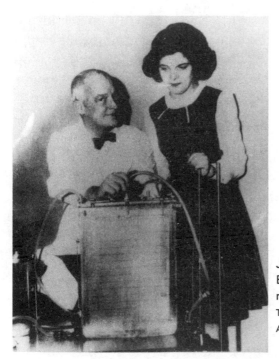

John Gibbon and Cecelia
Bavolek beside a heart-lung
machine, 1963 (Courtesy of
Thomas Jefferson University,
Archives and Special Collections)

chest, she was awake and could move her limbs on command. Her recovery was uneventful, and after thirteen days, she was discharged from the hospital. She went on to live for almost fifty years, dying in 2000 (the year before I started my cardiology training) at the age of sixty-five.

Though *Time* proclaimed that Gibbon had "made the dream [of open-heart surgery] a reality," he was painfully shy and avoided publicity. He posed for a picture with his machine only after Bavolek agreed to join him. In the end, he published the only account of his operation in a little-noticed journal, *Minnesota Medicine.*

After the Bavolek surgery, Gibbon attempted four more with his heart-lung machine, with poor results. Though his research career was marked by tremendous perseverance and courage, after those four children died under his knife, he lost heart. Unlike Walt Lillehei, who never lost sight of the greater goal, even in the face of surgical deaths, Gibbon could not stomach putting young children at risk, even if it meant giving up on his lifelong project. He decided that his machine was too immature to be used safely and called for a one-year moratorium on its use. He never operated on the heart again. Research on his machine was taken up by universities and private companies. In 1973, he died of a heart attack while playing tennis.

Today heart-lung machines are barely the size of a small refrigerator. Hospitals have full-time staff to operate them. Of course, there are still complications: blood cells get chewed up in the plastic and metal apparatus and patients suffer strokes. A small but significant number of patients have some degree of cognitive impairment afterward, such as memory and attention deficits and language problems, a condition known as "pump head," which can persist years after surgery and in many cases is probably irreversible. The cause is unclear but may include tiny blood clots or bubbles, inadequate blood flow to the brain during surgery, the dislodgement of fatty material from the aorta, and brain inflammation.

But despite these problems, the heart-lung machine has been indispensable for advancing the field of heart surgery over the past half century, saving countless lives. Open-heart surgery was already the beacon of American medical prowess in the early 1950s, and Gibbon's invention only quickened the field's progress. The mortality rate for cardiac surgery dropped from 50 percent in 1955, to 20 percent in 1956, to 10 percent in 1957. By the late 1950s, even the most complex congenital lesions were being repaired. "A physician at the bedside of a child dying of an intracardiac malformation as recently as 1952 could only pray for a recovery!" Lillehei wrote. "Today with the heart-lung machine, correction is routine." The heart became, as one writer put it, "an object of surgical assault."

Perhaps my own family history would have had a different trajectory had Gibbon's invention been ready for my grandfather, who surely had coronary artery disease and almost certainly died of a coronary thrombosis. Alas, the field would have to wait until 1960, when the first successful human coronary artery bypass operation was performed by Dr. Michael Rohman in the Bronx. In 1967, René Favaloro performed the world's first coronary bypass surgery at the Cleveland Clinic using veins from the leg to bypass the coronary obstructions, the standard technique still in use. Today more than one million cardiac operations are performed annually worldwide—three thousand a day—with the heart-lung machine.

•

One of those operations was that valve surgery in Fargo on Christmas Day. It had been going on for more than two hours when Dr. Shah finally cut out the infected valve with a pair of scissors. I'd been standing quietly next to him the whole time, my legs increasingly heavy and sore, wondering when the operation would end. Shah put green-and-yellow Gore-Tex threads, the same stuff in my winter jacket, through the cloth ring holding the prosthetic tissue valve. It was a mess, like the tangled ropes of a parachute, a topological nightmare, but when he slid the new valve down the circular array of stitches, the sutures straightened out and the valve went right into place.

When he was finished, he tipped the head of the table down so if there was any air in the heart, it would travel upward, away from the brain. The perfusionist turned a dial, and the flow of the heart-lung machine slowed. When Shah took the clamp off the aorta, blood started to flow down the coronaries, washing out the potassium solution that had made the heart fibrillate. The heart began to beat weakly, almost in synchrony with the labored breathing of the ventilator. Shah removed the remaining tubes from the chest. Then, with stainless-steel wires, his assistant closed up the breastbone.

We were done. I was so relieved, mostly for the patient but also, I must admit, because I wanted to go home. It was nearly five o'clock in the morning, and I could barely stand. But Shah looked worried. The patient's blood pressure was 70/40, dangerously low. The heart hadn't quite resumed adequate function. After conferring with the anesthesiologist, he inserted a helium-filled balloon pump into the aorta to support the blood pressure. With a pained expression, he sat down on a stool next to the still-unconscious patient and waited.

I waited, too, for a while, hoping something would happen so we could call it a night. By then Shah was ignoring me. I went to the locker room to change. Some time later, a nurse woke me up on the hard bench and told me she was going to take me home. We drove quickly along slushy roads coated with what looked like mashed potatoes and gravy. The sun was rising, and the trees along the road carried the weight of several inches of snow that had fallen during the night. She dropped me off at my parents' house. I went in and immediately crashed.

Shah never called me to tell me what happened, but the next day I heard from my parents that the patient never made it out of the OR. His blood pressure continued to drop, despite the balloon pump and intravenous medications, and around seven that morning, nearly seven hours after we'd arrived at the hospital, he died, another victim of endocarditis, Osler's great killer. It was an important lesson for me at that early stage in my career. No matter the extraordinary progress that has been made in heart surgery over the past century, the heart remains a vulnerable organ. Despite our best efforts, cardiac patients still die.

6

Nut

> The contemplation of the period when arterial disease of
> the heart can be prevented or retarded produces an aura
> of greatness. Next to food, shelter, and the absence of war,
> there is probably nothing more important.
> —Claude Beck, *Journal of Thoracic Surgery* (1958)

When I began my cardiology fellowship in 2001, the dingy catheterization labs at Bellevue looked as if they hadn't been renovated since André Cournand and Dickinson Richards did their seminal work on cardiac catheterization—a procedure used to measure pressures and flows in the heart's chambers and the coronary arteries—at Bellevue in the 1930s. The paint was peeling, lights had a dusty glow, and angiograms were still recorded on rolls of film—not digitized, as they were at the other major Manhattan teaching hospitals. Rhoda, the stern charge nurse, and her cadre of graying, droopy-lidded assistants— they, too, looked like artifacts of World War II. Rhoda would never tell you what she wanted you to do. It was a lot easier to yell at you after you made a mistake. My first month in the cath lab felt a lot like internship—except now I was in my thirties, married, and seven years into my medical education. If I asked whether a patient needed preoperative blood work, Rhoda or her assistants would act as if I were stupid or arrogant because it was in their protocol, and they had been doing it for years, and shouldn't I know this, and who was I to tell them what to do? There was so much to see to: take a history and examine the patient; X-rays, bloods, consent, and so on. The rhythm of the day got digitized into tiny to-do boxes, to be filled in at every hour. What motivated the long hours was fear: fear of overlooking something that could hurt a patient, of course, but more immediately fear of rebuke, of being dressed down for mismanagement or an oversight. And so I came to think of my cardiology training as being on dual tracks: learning *about* the heart, obviously, but also what was *in* my heart—what I was made of—at the same time.

Dr. Fuchs, the cath lab chief, didn't ease the tension any with his intimidating stare, his patronizing admonishments to dress like him (blue scrubs, white sneakers only), and his pompous talk of Henry Green and other obscure novelists. The first time I scrubbed in with him, Fuchs went rapid-fire through a series of instructions on how to operate the baffle, a small-keyboard-sized plastic contraption with an array of stopcocks attached to fluid-filled lines that was the nerve center of every catheterization procedure. My hands shook in a fine tremor as he ran through the different ways to open and close the stopcocks to flush the catheter, get rid of bubbles, inject X-ray-opaque dye into the coronary arteries, and so on. "Whatever you do," he said, tapping on a small white knob, "don't inject unless you turn this stopcock." Otherwise, he warned, a dangerous amount of pressure could build up in the catheter. A minute later, he advanced the catheter up the aorta, twisted it around the arch, and with some fine finger movements inserted it into the right coronary artery. "Okay, here we go," he said, moving the table up and down and side to side, adjusting the position just right under the camera. He stepped onto the fluoroscopy pedal, which controlled the X-ray source that would take pictures of the coronary arteries. It produced a crackling sound, like kindling catching fire. "Inject!" he boomed. I reflexively stepped onto the pedal that released dye. "Stop!" he shouted. "I told you never to do that!" I stood frozen, wondering what I had done wrong. He quickly turned the critical knob to relieve the excess pressure in the catheter. Then, ordering me away from the table, he put one foot on the fluoroscopy pedal and the other on the dye pedal and did the angiogram by himself.

It got easier. I didn't think it would, but it did. Lucas, a kind senior cardiology fellow, got me a baffle to practice on and methodically, professorially, went through all the knobs and combinations with which I should become familiar. Procedural cardiology, I quickly learned, was a craft; you got better with practice. I'd never been especially good with my hands, but after a few months I was able to do the first half of a cardiac catheterization on my own. The satisfaction I experienced doing an angiogram was something I'd never expected. The procedure became ritual: Lead apron, sterile gown, carefully arranging the instruments we were going to use with the precision of a sushi chef. Then a quick squirt of lidocaine to numb the groin. Needle finds the femoral artery. A burst of maroon fills the syringe. Blood spurts on the sterile drape (and sometimes the stone floor). Guide wire into the artery. Deep nick with a scalpel. Dilate the soft tissue to create a track for the catheter. Push, push. Blood gushing, don't panic. Catheter slips over the wire, connect it quickly to the baffle. Okay, deep breath, deep breath, here we go . . .

Like the heartbeat itself, catheterization was mechanical, repetitive; we performed more than a few every single day. Procedural comfort eventually lent a certain balance, confidence, to my fellowship experience. For the first time that I could remember, physical action alleviated my anxiety, providing me with a zone of calmness in which to operate. When I was doing a cath, the world outside disappeared for just a few minutes. The procedure, with me as conductor, was all that mattered. In the cath lab, I was a doer, a craftsman, and not just a thinker. Seeing a plastic tube inside the heart quickly ceased to shock, which, in the end, was the most shocking thing of all.

•

For most of history, inserting anything like a catheter into the human heart was considered madness. But things changed on a hot May afternoon in 1929, when a surgical intern named Werner Forssmann and a nurse named Gerda Ditzen tiptoed into an operating room at the Auguste-Viktoria Hospital in Eberswalde, Germany, a small town fifty miles northwest of Berlin. For more than a week, they had been planning a tryst, but not of the carnal kind. Quietly closing the door behind them, Forssmann ordered Ditzen onto a surgical table, where he tied her down, immobilizing her arm. Sweating profusely in the heat, she anxiously awaited his long scalpel, believing, as Forssmann had told her, that she was going to be the subject of an experiment that would change the course of medicine. But

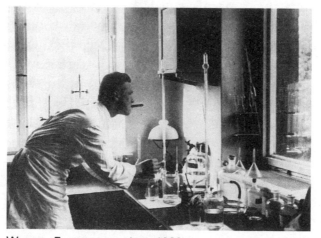

Werner Forssmann, circa 1928 (Courtesy of *The American Journal of Cardiology* 79, no. 5 [1997])

Forssmann had a different plan. Turning his back to her, he applied antiseptic soap to his own arm and quickly injected anesthetic into the skin and soft tissue. Then, armed with a scalpel, he sliced open the skin over his elbow pit with an inch-long incision. Droplets of fat and blood, like clusters of tiny grapes, followed the track of his blade.

Nothing in Forssmann's background could have predicted such brazen, almost criminal action. He was born in Berlin on August 29, 1904, the only child of a lawyer and a home-maker. Blond and blue-eyed, he was raised in a Prussian household with Prussian rules and a Prussian respect for law and order. His father was killed in battle during World War I, leaving his mother and grandmother (a woman he affection-ately referred to as "old corset bone," because she was so rigid) to supervise his early education. However, it was his uncle Walter, a small-town physician with whom Forssmann made house calls in a yellow two-horse carriage, who encouraged him to study medicine. His hard-nosed uncle did not tolerate squeamishness. He once made the teenage Forssmann go to the local prison to cut down a prisoner who'd hanged himself in his cell.

In 1922, seven years before his tryst with Ditzen, the eighteen-year-old Forssmann entered medical school at the University of Berlin. In his first year, he was nauseated by ani-mal experiments; like many, the wobbly youth did not enjoy pithing frogs. In the anatomy lab, Forssmann later recalled, a professor once joked that "the only way to a woman's heart is through her vagina. You go from the uterus and the Fallo-pian tubes to the abdominal cavity, then via the lymphatic space into the lymphatic vessels and veins and thus to the goal!" Perhaps this, Forssmann cheekily wrote, is what inspired him in his later attempts to reach the heart through the vascular system.

In his first year in medical school, Forssmann became fascinated with the heart, particularly the experiments of the

French scientist Claude Bernard, widely considered the father of modern experimental physiology. Bernard measured pressure in the cardiac chambers of horses and other animals by inserting rubber catheters through blood vessels and into their hearts. (In fact, he coined the term "cardiac catheterization.") Bernard's animal studies convinced Forssmann that inserting a catheter into a human heart would also be safe. The young medical student wanted to check the heart's pressures and flows, to understand and operationalize its basic functions, as one would a complex machine. No doubt he wanted to expunge the heart of its emotional connotations. But the idea that the human heart was just a pump, like an animal's, was still anathema.

After graduating in the spring of 1928, Forssmann joined the surgical staff at the Auguste-Viktoria Hospital in Eberswalde. Not long after beginning his internship, Forssmann mentioned his interest in cardiac catheterization to his chief, Richard Schneider, a modest and reserved administrator who was also a Forssmann family friend. The young intern described an audacious plan to insert a thin, flexible tube into a vein and advance it along the superior vena cava and into the right side of the heart. Moreover, he wanted to do this on a living person: himself. Schneider immediately nixed the plan. The human heart was an inviolable sanctuary; invading it with a foreign object was a medical and cultural taboo. Like most mid-level academic administrators, Schneider had no appetite for such adventure. "Remember your mother," the chief cried. "Imagine how it would be if I had to inform this lady, who has already lost her husband, that her only son had died in my hospital as a result of an experiment which I had approved." However, Schneider was reluctant to discourage Forssmann completely. He suggested trying the procedure on animals first.

But Forssmann—brash, ambitious, and naive to the ways of academia—did not drop the idea. He persuaded a fellow intern,

Peter Romeis, to help him perform the experiment. A week before his jaunt with Nurse Ditzen, the story goes, he met Romeis in an operating room at the hospital. With his colleague's assistance, Forssmann made an incision in his left arm and inserted a rubber bladder catheter into the antecubital vein, which drains blood from the hand. Unfortunately, the thirty-five-centimeter catheter wasn't long enough to reach the heart. (The typical distance from hand to heart in an adult is sixty to eighty centimeters.) When Forssmann insisted on walking to the fluoroscopy lab to take an X-ray to document the catheter's position, Romeis panicked and yanked the catheter out.* He later said that he'd always found Forssmann to be "a rather queer, peculiar person, lone and desolate, hardly ever mingling with his coworkers socially. One never knew whether he was thinking or mentally deficient."

Though the practice has been largely hidden, self-experimentation in medicine has a long history. Through the centuries, as the journalist Lawrence Altman has detailed, doctors and scientists have often decided to do research first on themselves. Some have done so for moral reasons, wanting to assume an experiment's risk before imposing it on others. There were also practical considerations: identifying subjects to participate in research isn't always easy. In the eighteenth century, for example, John Hunter, physician to King George III, intentionally injected his own penis with the purulent discharge of a patient with gonorrhea to investigate the transmission of that disease, contracting both gonorrhea *and* syphilis (the patient apparently had both). A hundred years later, Daniel Carrión, a medical student in Lima, injected himself with the blood of a boy with *verruga peruana*, then a common disorder in Peru, to prove that *verruga* and "Oroya fever" were manifestations of the same

*Forssmann told the journalist Lawrence Altman that this story, which Forssmann himself publicized, was apocryphal.

infection. Carrión fell into a coma and died thirty-nine days later.

Whatever Forssmann's motivations, he eventually sweet-talked Ditzen, the surgical nurse who held the keys to the supply closet, into getting him a longer catheter, prowling around her "like a sweet-toothed cat around the cream jug," as he later wrote. A week later, on the afternoon of May 12, 1929, while his colleagues napped in their call rooms, he was ready to try again. Ditzen believed she was going to be Forssmann's first subject. Forssmann had a different idea.

After slicing open the skin over the elbow crease of his left arm, Forssmann widened the wound with metal forceps to get a better view. He dissected down to the antecubital vein, periodically dabbing the oozing blood to clear the view. He pulled the vein up taut to the skin surface; it had the color and consistency of an earthworm. He must have tied off the vein upstream from where he was going to cut to minimize bleeding. Then he transected the vein. It quickly drained of blood, collapsing on itself like a flimsy membrane. Forssmann inserted the sixty-five-centimeter catheter provided by Ditzen into the hole and advanced it. He later said that he experienced a warm sensation as the flexible tube scraped along the walls of his veins, as well as a slight cough, which he attributed to stimulation of the vagus, the main parasympathetic nerve in the body. With the catheter dangling out of his bleeding arm, he released Ditzen, who had apparently been protesting and struggling to get free, and ordered the angry nurse to follow him to the fluoroscopy lab to help him take a picture. Perhaps realizing they were about to make history—or maybe out of fear of the self-butchering intern—Ditzen acquiesced. They slipped downstairs. In the fluoroscopy lab, Forssmann lay down on a stretcher, while Ditzen held a mirror in front of him so that he could observe the catheter tip on a camera screen. The first X-ray showed that the catheter had not yet reached its destination, so Forssmann pushed it even farther until his arm had swallowed nearly all of it. In the middle of all this, Romeis, Forssmann's colleague, hair tousled and still half-asleep, burst into the fluoroscopy lab and tried to stop Forssmann. Apparently, the word around the hospital was that Forssmann was trying to commit suicide. Romeis found Forssmann silent and pale on a gurney, sheets soaked with blood, catheter still in his arm, staring up at the ceiling. "What the hell are you doing?" he cried. Forssmann wrote that he had to give Romeis "a few kicks in the shin to calm him down." As Forssmann pushed in the last few centimeters, the catheter tip clearly passed under his armpit and into the right atrium. It was a seminal moment—a violation, really—that philosophers and physicians had awaited—indeed feared—for centuries. Ditzen and a flabbergasted radiology technician snapped a photograph to document the catheter's position. Then Forssmann pulled the tube out of his body.

When he learned what Forssmann had done, Schneider was incensed at the disobedience, even as he acknowledged (over drinks at a nearby tavern) that Forssmann had made an important contribution to medical science. "Say that you tried it on cadavers before you did it on yourself," Schneider urged, hoping to keep Forssmann from appearing like a nut to the scientific community. In any case, there was nothing at Eberswalde for his protégé. He suggested Forssmann transfer to a more research-oriented facility to pursue his interests.

A few months later, Forssmann took an unpaid position at the Charité Hospital in Berlin. In November 1929, his self-experiment was published in *Klinische Wochenschrift*, a leading journal. The paper, "Probing the Right Ventricle of the Heart," received widespread press coverage, but Forssmann was ridiculed as a quack in the medical world. There were no obvious applications of his procedure—this would change within a few years—and Forssmann's fanciful proposal to use cardiac catheterization for metabolic studies or cardiac resuscitation did not gain him any supporters. Moreover, Ernst Unger, a

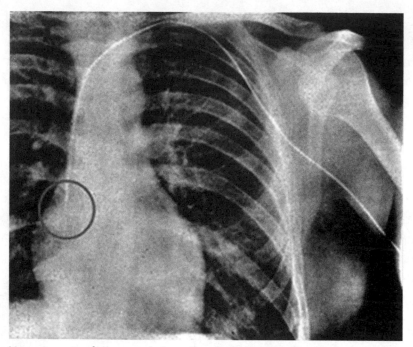

X-ray image of Forssmann's self-catheterization, showing a catheter
threaded through his arm and into his right atrium (*circled*) (Reproduced
by permission; from W. Forssmann, *Klinische Wochenschrift* 8 [1929]: 2085–87)

leading German surgeon, falsely claimed that he had already
performed cardiac catheterization many years before and that
Forssmann had not properly acknowledged his work, a claim
that was repudiated by *Klinische*'s editor. With controversy
swirling around him, Forssmann, just twenty-six years old, was
fired. His chairman, Ferdinand Sauerbruch, one of the leading
academic surgeons in Germany, reportedly told him, "You qualify to work in a circus, not in a reputable clinic."

In January 1930, Schneider allowed Forssmann to return
to Eberswalde, where the young doctor resumed his catheter
experiments. He finally performed animal studies, keeping experimental dogs at his mother's apartment, where he would inject them with morphine, put them in a sack, and lug them to
the hospital on his motorcycle. Over the following year, Forss-

mann did more experiments on himself, too, injecting opaque dye into his own heart to better visualize its function under X-ray. Though the pictures were poor and his experiments largely unsuccessful, Forssmann kept going until he had scarred all the usable veins in his arms (as well as butchered a few in his groin). Despite the sacrifices to his body, at surgical conferences Forssmann's talks would be placed last on the agenda and received little attention. Discouraged by the lack of progress and his work's chilly reception, Forssmann abandoned cardiology and turned to urology. He eventually went into private practice, like his uncle Walter, in a small town in the Black Forest.

Forssmann's self-experiments did not go unnoticed, however. In the late 1930s, two American scientists, André Cournand and Dickinson Richards, working at Columbia-Presbyterian Medical Center and later at Bellevue Hospital in New York City, came across Forssmann's techniques and applied them to measure cardiac pressures and flows, first in dogs and chimpanzees and later in humans. With war looming, their work was encouraged by the federal government's interest in supporting research on blood circulation that could help in the treatment of traumatic shock. Over a ten-year period, the Bellevue scientists used modified bladder catheters just millimeters in diameter to study the dynamics of blood flow in patients with congenital, pericardial, and rheumatic heart disease. American cardiology was brought into the modern age.*

In 1956, nearly three decades after Forssmann's seminal experiment, Cournand, Richards, and Forssmann shared the Nobel Prize in Physiology or Medicine "for their discoveries concerning heart catheterization and pathological changes in

*Progress was slower abroad. John McMichael, a doctor in London, wanted to use catheterization in his own shock study. He contacted Cournand, who shared information on the technique. However, a colleague of McMichael's warned him that the technique was dangerous and that he would not be defended in court if he was charged with manslaughter if a patient died.

the circulatory system." In his Nobel lecture, Cournand paid homage to Forssmann, stating that the cardiac catheter was "the key in the lock" to discover the intricate physiology of the human heart. Indeed, cardiac catheterization was undoubtedly one of the greatest medical discoveries of the twentieth century, ushering in numerous applications, such as coronary angiography, coronary stenting, and right-heart studies, that have saved countless from premature deaths. For his part, Forssmann declared that he felt "like a village parson who has just learned that he has been made bishop." Despite the Nobel Prize, he never returned to cardiac research, however. "The subject had progressed too far," he wrote, "and when I considered it objectively I was certain I'd never catch up." He decided "it was more honest to content myself with the role of leading fossil." Forssmann continued his private urology practice. On June 1, 1979, he died of a heart attack.

Within a decade after Forssmann's epoch-making experiment, the taboo about touching the heart had been demolished. Scientists explored every avenue of access to animal and human hearts—under the breastbone; through the ribs; just below the nipple; through the left atrium; through the aorta; through the suprasternal notch, the soft spot above the breastbone and below the throat; and even through the back—giving them unprecedented access to the physiology of a once mysterious organ.

But as is so often the case in science, once the taboo about touching the heart was breached, it was transformed into something equally inviolable. Accessing the heart's apple-sized chambers was one thing. Inserting needles into the coronary arteries that supply blood to those chambers was a different challenge altogether. Coronary arteries are small, hardly five millimeters in diameter. When they are diseased with fatty plaque, their diameter can shrink to microns. No one thought that dye could be safely injected into these vessels because it was feared that occluding a coronary artery with a catheter for even a few seconds would precipitate a fatal arrhythmia. Even the fearless Forssmann never messed with the coronaries; they were only studied at autopsy. Though animal studies did not validate doctors' widespread fears, the human heart was once again believed to be uniquely impervious to intervention. But did it have to remain so? After World War II, the coronary arteries became the new frontier in cardiac medicine, and the holy grail.

7

Stress Fractures

Every affection of the mind that is attended either with
pain or pleasure, hope or fear, is the cause of an agitation
whose influence extends to the heart.
—William Harvey, *De Motu Cordis* (1628)

In the catheterization lab, I was able to visualize the
consequences—stony plaque, obstructive clot—of coronary artery disease. But why did the disease develop in the first place?
This was a question that vexed scientists at mid century, even as
the heart-lung machine was being developed and cardiac catheterization techniques were being refined. (As is so often true
in medicine, treatment outpaced understanding.) But by the
1960s, doctors had an idea—albeit incomplete—of the answer.
And it came from a study begun in a small town in Massachusetts shortly after World War II that almost single-handedly
defines the modern science of heart disease.

The impetus for the Framingham Heart Study was obvious.
In the 1940s, cardiovascular disease was the main cause of mortality in the United States, accounting for nearly half of all
deaths. However, what was known about heart disease wasn't
enough to fill even a slim chapter in a modern textbook.

Doctors, for example, did not know that myocardial infarction was caused by total or near-total obstruction of a coronary artery. (This mechanism wasn't even mentioned in popular literature until 1955, when Humbert Humbert in *Lolita* is said to die of a "coronary thrombosis.") The jury was also out on whether angina, chest pain caused by decreased coronary blood flow, was a psychological syndrome or a disease based on an organic cause. "Prevention and treatment were so poorly understood," Dr. Thomas Wang and his colleagues wrote in *The Lancet* a few years ago, "that most Americans accepted early death from heart disease as unavoidable."

One who fell victim to this ignorance was our thirty-second president. Franklin Delano Roosevelt was in poor health for much of his presidency, even though his doctors, his family, and even journalists colluded to portray him as the picture of health. (Few in the public knew, for example, that Roosevelt was essentially confined to a wheelchair after contracting polio when he was thirty-nine.) Roosevelt's personal physician, Admiral Ross McIntire, an ear, nose, and throat specialist, seemed to hardly pay attention to the president's blood pressure as it rose over his four terms. When Roosevelt began his second term in 1937, his blood pressure was 170/100 (normal today is considered less than 140/90). When the Japanese bombed Pearl Harbor in 1941, it was 190/105. By the time American soldiers landed in Normandy in June 1944, it was 226/118, life-threateningly high. At the Yalta Conference in February 1945, Winston Churchill's doctor wrote that Roosevelt "has all the symptoms of hardening of the arteries" and "I give him only a few months to live." Yet McIntire insisted that the president was healthy and that his problems were "no more than normal for a man of his age."*

Within a month of Roosevelt's last State of the Union ad-

*The British were under no such delusions. When Churchill visited the White House in May 1943, he asked his own physician whether he had noticed that

dress, in which he declared that "1945 can be the greatest year of achievement in human history," his condition had visibly deteriorated. Roosevelt had already been admitted to Bethesda Naval Hospital with shortness of breath, profuse sweating, and abdominal swelling: classic signs of congestive heart failure. Howard Bruenn, one of only a few hundred cardiologists in the country at the time, gave the president a diagnosis of "hypertensive heart disease and cardiac failure." However, there were few treatments available to him. He put Roosevelt on digitalis and a salt-restricted diet, but Roosevelt's blood pressure continued to rise. It remained life-threateningly high until April 12, 1945, when Roosevelt died at the age of sixty-three from a stroke and brain hemorrhage. His last words, sitting for a portrait in Warm Springs, Georgia, where he had gone to rehabilitate, were "I have a terrific headache."

Though it was a national tragedy, Roosevelt's death was not in vain. In 1948, Congress passed the National Heart Act, declaring "the Nation's health [to be] seriously threatened by diseases of the heart and circulation." Signing the bill into law, President Harry Truman called heart disease "our most challenging public health problem." The law established the National Heart Institute (NHI) within the National Institutes of Health to promote research into the prevention and treatment of cardiovascular disease. One of the first grants was for an epidemiological study to be conducted by the U.S. Public Health Service.

Epidemiology is about the ecology of disease: where and when it is found, or not. In 1854, John Snow, physician to Queen Victoria, performed the world's first epidemiological study when he investigated a major cholera outbreak in London's Soho district. Snow was born in the town of York, at the intersection of two rivers contaminated by dung and sewage.

Roosevelt was "a very tired man." He added, ominously, "The Americans here cannot bring themselves to believe that he is finished."

His childhood likely sensitized him to a community's need for clean water. Based on studies nearly ten years before the Soho epidemic, Snow had concluded that cholera was transmitted by "morbid matter," not foul air, as his colleagues at the London Medical Society believed. He based his theory in part on the fact that workers in slaughterhouses, thought to be a font of cholera, were afflicted no more than the general population. So, when cholera broke out in London in 1854, Snow set his sights on a well. He went to the General Registry Office and mapped the addresses of all the cholera deaths in the Soho district, discovering that most deaths had occurred near a water pump on Broad Street. True to his meticulous nature, Snow also studied Soho residents who did not contract the disease—for example, inmates at a nearby prison that did not use the Broad Street pump, as well as brewery workers whose supervisor, a Mr. Huggins, told Snow that his men drank only water from the brewery's own well (when they weren't consuming the malt liquor they produced).

Though Snow knew nothing of germs, he was nevertheless able to contain the epidemic, which caused 616 deaths, by persuading the board of governors of the local parish to remove the handle on the well's pump, making it impossible to draw water. Only later, by studying water samples, did London authorities show that the pump was contaminated with sewage from a nearby cesspool, setting off what Snow called "the most terrible outbreak of cholera which ever occurred in this kingdom." Snow's investigation saved many lives. Just as important, it showed that an epidemic could be controlled without a precise understanding of its cause.*

After Snow's study and the subsequent development of epidemiological techniques, public health authorities in the United States focused their attention on acute infectious diseases like

*Thirty years later, in 1884, Robert Koch, a German physician, isolated the pathogen *Vibrio cholerae*, which causes cholera.

cholera, tuberculosis, and leprosy. Chronic noninfectious ailments—the long-term hard hitters like heart disease—received little attention. But after Roosevelt's death, Assistant Surgeon General Joseph Mountin, a founder of the Office of Malaria Control in War Areas (later known as the Centers for Disease Control, or CDC), was eager to correct this disparity. As was the case with cholera in the mid-nineteenth century, very little was known about the determinants of heart disease. Could risk factors be identified by studying people who developed the disease, just as Snow had studied the victims of the cholera epidemic?

The national climate after World War II was favorable for such an investigation. New hospitals were being built, the National Institutes of Health was expanding, and there was increased federal commitment to basic and clinical research. Moreover, a beloved president had just died. In this environment, things moved quickly. By the summer of 1948, the U.S. Public Health Service had already negotiated the basic framework of an epidemiological study of heart disease with the Massachusetts Department of Health. The commonwealth was a natural choice for the project, with top medical schools, such as Harvard, Tufts, and the University of Massachusetts, in and around Boston. The commissioner of health was "warmly enthusiastic" about a pilot study to develop heart-screening tools. With the support of Harvard physicians, the town of Framingham, about twenty miles west of Boston, was chosen as the site.

In the late seventeenth century, Framingham was a farming community, home of the first teachers' college and the first women's prison, and a haven for those trying to escape the witch hunts in nearby Salem. During the Civil War, it was the first town in Massachusetts to establish a volunteer battalion. However, by the 1940s, Framingham had turned into a middle-class industrial town. Children played with garden hoses on tree-lined streets. The 28,000 townsfolk lived mostly in single-family homes and earned a median family income of about $5,000 per year (about $50,000 today). (There were exceptions, of course, such as James Roosevelt, the president's son, who owned a large estate on Salem End Road.) Most Framingham residents ate a typical meat-and-potatoes diet. Like the rest of the country, about half of them smoked. Predominantly white and of western European descent, they were believed to be representative of America after World War II.

The key question at the heart of the Framingham study was this: Can the risk of a heart attack be predicted in a person with no overt heart disease? The plan was to follow approximately five thousand healthy patients between the ages of thirty and fifty-nine for twenty years until enough of them developed heart disease. Meanwhile, factors associated with the development of the disease would be identified (and later, hopefully, modified to prevent disease in healthy patients). At the time, hypothetical factors were "nervous and mental states," occupation, economic status, and use of stimulants like Benzedrine. Though research linking heart disease with cholesterol had been available for decades (in 1913, researchers in St. Petersburg had demonstrated that feeding rabbits large quantities of cholesterol-rich foods, such as meat and eggs, caused atherosclerotic plaques), this information was not yet widely known to doctors or the American public.

The initial outlay for the Framingham study was modest: about $94,000, mostly to cover office supplies (including ashtrays for the study researchers who smoked). Mountin, the assistant surgeon general, selected Gilcin Meadors, a young U.S. Public Health Service officer, as the first director. Born in Mississippi, Meadors had graduated from medical school at Tulane only eight years earlier. When he was tapped by Mountin, he was still completing a master's degree in public health at Johns Hopkins. Besides a lack of experience, Meadors faced many challenges. He had to persuade local physicians, many of them suspicious of the federal government, to cooperate with the U.S. Public Health Service. Moreover, because of the long period required for heart disease to develop in healthy people, nearly half the eligible townsfolk would have to agree to participate, and their attrition rate would have to be almost vanishingly low.

The study was announced in a small advertisement in the local newspaper on October 11, 1948. Then Meadors, the young upstart epidemiologist, went into action. Not your typical pocket-protector bureaucrat, Meadors was charming and sociable. He attended town meetings and befriended civic leaders. Flattered by his ambition, a whole network of veterans, lawyers, and housewives sprang up to spread word about the study. Meadors's recruits knocked on doors, staffed telephone banks, and appeared at churches, parent-teacher organizations, and community groups. Their mission was to help him enroll subjects willing to reveal intimate information to federal officials with no promise of any direct benefit (though Meadors said the study would eventually lead to "recommendations for the modification of personal habits and environment"). Within weeks, Meadors's staff had filled appointment slots through the spring.

The first study questionnaires included items about personal and family history, parents' age at the time of death, habits, mental state, and medication use. Government-appointed doctors peered into subjects' eyes and palpated livers and lymph nodes. Blood and urine tests were taken; X-rays and electrocardiograms were performed. Though cholesterol testing had been considered before the initiation of the study, it was only added after the research had begun.

After a year, control of the study shifted to the newly established National Heart Institute. The NHI changed the character of the project, making its methodology more rigorous. Instead of enrolling volunteers, it now randomly selected subjects, eliminating a source of bias. The focus also shifted toward investigating biological rather than "psychosocial" risk factors. Questions about sexual dysfunction, psychiatric problems, emotional stress, income, and social class were discarded. Statisticians at the NHI invented something called multivariate analysis, a method of calculating the relative importance of each of several factors that coexist in the expression of a disease. (In the beginning, Framingham scientists focused on age, serum cholesterol, weight, electrocardiographic abnormalities, red blood cell count, number of cigarettes smoked, and systolic blood pressure.) Therefore, the Framingham study, as it emerged in the 1950s, was "clinically narrow," as one researcher put it, "with little interest in investigating psychosomatic, constitutional, or sociological determinants of heart disease." This would turn out to be a major flaw.

After nearly ten years of closely monitoring approximately fifty-two hundred patients, Framingham researchers published a key paper in 1957 (out of the nearly three thousand produced to date) showing that patients with high blood pressure had a nearly fourfold increase in the incidence of coronary heart disease. A few years later, hypertension was also shown to be a major cause of stroke. Referring to President Roosevelt's premature death, Framingham scientists commented on the "mounting evidence that many of the commonly accepted beliefs concerning hypertension and its cardiovascular consequences may be in error." Even Dr. Bruenn, Roosevelt's cardiologist, wrote, "I have often wondered what turn the subsequent course of history might have taken if the modern methods for the control of hypertension had been available."

Later Framingham publications identified additional coronary risk factors, including diabetes and high serum cholesterol. One paper found that nearly one in five heart attacks present with sudden death as the first and only symptom, a discovery that ratified the tremendous fear that millions of Americans were living with. By the early 1960s, a definitive association had also been made between cigarette smoking and heart disease. (Smokers in previous studies hadn't lived long enough to draw definitive conclusions.) This led to the first surgeon general's report detailing the health hazards of smoking. In 1966, the United States became the first country to require warning labels on cigarette packages. Four years later, primarily because of Framingham, President Nixon signed legislation banning cigarette ads on television and radio, one of the great public health triumphs of the second half of the twentieth century.

The Framingham study was nearly shut down in the late 1960s for lack of funding. There was no dearth of events— assassinations, riots, civil rights protests, and the Vietnam War—to occupy policy makers, and an epidemiological study in a small town in Massachusetts hardly seemed to warrant much attention. So, Framingham investigators went around the country trying to raise private money. Donors included some unexpected contributors, including the Tobacco Institute and the Oscar Mayer Company, which manufactured luncheon meats. In the end, only after President Nixon's personal physician, the cardiologist Paul Dudley White, lobbied for the study was federal support revived.

The Framingham study shifted the focus of medicine from treating cardiovascular disease to preventing it in those at risk. (Indeed, the term "risk factor" was introduced by Framingham researchers in 1961.) In 1998, while I was still in medical school, Framingham researchers published a formula, based on the major independent cardiac risk factors that had been identified— family history, smoking, diabetes, high serum cholesterol, and hypertension—to calculate a patient's risk of getting heart disease within ten years. (This is the formula I used after my first CT scan showing that I had developed coronary plaque.) Today we know that programs that target such risk factors improve public health. For example, a recent twelve-year study of 20,000 Swedish men showed that almost four out of five heart attacks could be prevented through Framingham-inspired lifestyle changes, such as a healthy diet, moderate alcohol consumption, no smoking, increased physical activity, and maintaining a normal body weight. Men who adopted all five changes were

86 percent less likely to have a heart attack than those who did not. An earlier study of about 88,000 young female nurses found that participants who followed a healthy lifestyle—didn't smoke, had normal body weight, exercised at least two and a half hours each week, had moderate alcohol consumption, followed a healthy diet, and watched little television—had almost no heart disease after twenty years of follow-up.

But as important as the Framingham Heart Study has been in advancing our understanding of coronary heart disease, it does not tell the whole story. For example, Framingham risk models do not seem to apply equally to nonwhite ethnic groups. Meadors and the early Framingham investigators recognized the lack of diversity in the study population as a major limitation.* What of my medical school cadaver or my grandfather? In 1959, the first study showing an increased risk of premature heart disease in Indian males was published in *The American Heart Journal*. These men had four times the rate of heart disease compared with men living in Framingham, despite having lower rates of hypertension, smoking, and high cholesterol and more often consuming a vegetarian diet. Today in South Asia, a large percentage of heart attacks occur in men with zero or only one Framingham risk factor. Over the past half century, coronary artery disease rates have increased threefold in urban India and twofold in rural India. During that time, the average age at which a first heart attack occurs has increased by ten years in the United States but decreased by about ten years in India. Compared with whites, South Asians have more multivessel coronary artery disease and are more likely to have a more dangerous anterior location of a myocardial infarction. South Asians will soon make up over half of the world's cardiac patients. What is it about South Asian genetics

---

*In later years, Framingham investigators added about a thousand ethnic minority patients to their study to try to understand why heart disease occurs disproportionately in certain groups and to identify novel risk factors.

or environments that leads to so much heart disease? We need a Framingham-type study to answer this question.*

But there are almost certainly cardiovascular risk factors that Framingham investigators did not identify. Some of these factors are likely in the "psychosocial" domain that Framingham investigators decided to ignore when the study was taken over by the NHI in the early 1950s. For example, consider heart disease in Japanese immigrants. Coronary artery disease is relatively rare in Japan. However, its rate is almost double in Japanese immigrants who settle in Hawaii and triple in those who settle in the mainland United States. Part of the explanation might be that Japanese immigrants adopt unhealthy American habits, like a sedentary lifestyle or a diet rich in processed foods. Still, Framingham risk factors do not fully explain the disparity.

In the early 1970s, Sir Michael Marmot and his colleagues at the UC Berkeley School of Public Health studied nearly four thousand middle-aged Japanese men living in the San Francisco Bay Area. They found that immigrants who stayed true to their Japanese roots (as evidenced in surveys by their ability to read Japanese, the frequency with which they spoke Japanese, the frequency with which they had Japanese co-workers, and so on) had a much lower prevalence of heart disease, even when they matched Americans in terms of serum cholesterol and blood pressure, than immigrants who were more integrated into their new culture. "Traditional" Japanese immigrants had coronary disease rates in line with their homeland counterparts. "West-

---

*The National Institutes of Health has started such a study. Named Mediators of Atherosclerosis in South Asians Living in America, or MASALA, it has enrolled about nine hundred South Asian men and women in two large metropolitan areas, the San Francisco Bay Area and Chicago. Researchers are focusing on novel risk factors, including malignant forms of cholesterol (previous research has suggested that South Asians may have smaller and denser cholesterol particles that are more prone to causing hardening of the arteries), as well as other social, cultural, and genetic determinants.

ernized" immigrants had a prevalence that was at least three times higher. "Retention of Japanese group relationships is associated with a lower rate of coronary heart disease," the authors concluded. And so, acculturation, they declared, is a major risk factor for coronary disease in immigrant populations.

If cutting traditional cultural ties increases the risk of heart disease, then psychosocial factors must play a role in cardiovascular health. Today we know this to be true in many strata of human society. For example, American blacks in poor urban centers have a much higher prevalence of hypertension and cardiovascular disease than other groups. Some have proposed genetics to be the deciding factor; however, this is an unlikely explanation, because American blacks have hypertension at much higher rates than their West African counterparts. Moreover, hypertension pervades other segments of American society in which poverty and social ills are rampant.

Peter Sterling, the University of Pennsylvania neurobiologist, has written that hypertension in such communities is a normal response to what he calls "chronic arousal," or stress. In small preindustrial communities, he writes, people tend to know and trust one another. Generosity is rewarded; cheating tends to be punished. When this milieu is disrupted, as in migration or urbanization, there is often an increased need for vigilance. People get estranged from their neighbors. Communities become diverse and more mistrustful. Physical and social isolation often results. Add in poverty, fragmented families, and joblessness, and you get extremely stress-prone populations. The chronic arousal triggers release of hormones, such as adrenaline and cortisol, that tighten blood vessels and cause retention of salt. These in turn lead to long-term changes like arterial wall thickening and stiffening that increase the blood pressure that the body tries to maintain.

In Sterling's formulation, nothing is broken (except perhaps "the system"). The body is responding exactly in the way it should to the chronic fight-or-flight circumstances in which it finds itself. If takotsubo cardiomyopathy proves that acute psychological disruption can damage the heart, Sterling's theories suggest that chronic, low-level stress may be just as harmful. His theories put psychosocial factors front and center in how we think about and approach heart problems. They show that chronic heart disease, unloosed from a Framingham cage, is inextricably linked to the state of our neighborhoods, jobs, and families. Heart disease, in this conception, is no longer strictly biological; it is cultural and political as well. Improving our social structures and relationships becomes not only a quality-of-life issue but also a public health concern.*

The harmful cardiovascular effects of chronic arousal apply to traditionally white communities, too. One example is the Whitehall study, also conducted by Marmot, of seventeen thousand male workers in the British civil service. In this study, early death and poor health were found to increase stepwise

---

*Sterling's theory, allostasis, is a new way to think about human physiology. The traditional theory taught in medical school, homeostasis, holds that organ systems work together to maintain physiological balance. For example, when blood pressure drops acutely, the heart speeds up and the kidneys retain sodium and water, propelling blood pressure back to normal. If body temperature falls, we shiver to generate heat, blood vessels constrict to conserve heat, and we warm up. Homeostasis is about preserving constancy in the face of changing conditions. As a model for explaining human physiology, it does pretty well.

However, there are aspects of the human condition that homeostasis cannot explain. For instance, blood pressure often fluctuates minute to minute. If the body is supposed to be maintaining an optimal set point, it doesn't seem to be doing a very good job. Blood pressure also increases steadily throughout childhood and adulthood. It is often constant until about age six, when children enter school, but then it rises quickly as kids detach from their parents and must become vigilant at defending against real or perceived threats. By age seventeen, almost half of all boys have blood pressures in the pre-hypertensive range, and about 20 percent have full-blown hypertension. Why does the blood pressure set point drift upward? To explain these things, experts like Sterling have proposed an alternative theory to homeostasis: allostasis.

Allostasis is not about preserving constancy; it is about calibrating the body's functions in response to external as well as internal conditions. The body doesn't so much defend a particular set point as allow it to fluctuate in response to changing demands, including those of one's social circumstances. Allostasis is, in that sense, a politically sophisticated theory of human physiology. Indeed, because of its sensitivity to social circumstances, allostasis is in many ways better than homeostasis for explaining modern chronic diseases.

from the highest to the lowest levels of the civil service hierarchy. Messengers and porters had nearly twice the death rate of higher-ranking administrators, even after accounting for differences in smoking, plasma cholesterol, blood pressure, and alcohol consumption. None of these civil servants were poor, in the usual sense. They all enjoyed clean water, plenty of food, and proper toilet facilities. The main ways they differed were in occupational prestige, job control, and other gradients of the social hierarchy. Marmot and his co-workers concluded that emotional disturbance, because of financial instability, time pressures, lack of advancement, and a general dearth of autonomy, drives much of the difference in survival. "Both low-grade civil servant and slum dweller lack control over their lives," Marmot writes. "They do not have the opportunity to lead lives they have reason to value."

Lower socioeconomic classes are not the only ones susceptible to stress-induced heart problems. In the mid-1950s, Meyer Friedman and Ray Rosenman, two American cardiologists working at Mount Zion Hospital in San Francisco, created the idea of a high-achieving personality, which they called type A, that was particularly susceptible to heart disease and was disproportionately found in higher socioeconomic groups. "The type-A person is invariably punctual and greatly annoyed if kept waiting," they wrote. "He rarely finds time to indulge in hobbies, and when he does, he makes them as competitive as his vocation. He dislikes helping at home in routine jobs because he feels that his time can be spent more profitably. He walks rapidly, eats rapidly, and rarely remains long at the dinner table. He often tries to do several things at once." They described a characteristic physiognomy of this personality type. "[The type A man] tends to look you straight and quite unflinchingly in the eye. His face looks extraordinarily alert; that is, his eyes are very much alive, quickly seeking to take in the situation at a glance. He may employ a tense teeth-clenching and jaw-grinding posture. His smile has a lateral extension, and his laughter is rarely a 'belly-laugh.' " In short, they said, the type A person is "aggressively involved in a chronic, incessant struggle to achieve more and more in less and less time."

Friedman and Rosenman's research was girded by the idea "that a person's feelings and thoughts have an influence on the development of coronary heart disease." They wrote, "Too many finely executed studies suggested that neither cholesterol nor the fat content of various diets could always explain coronary heart disease. Other factors just had to be playing a part." In one of their studies, men who fit the type A pattern were seven times more likely to develop arterial disease than was a cohort of (presumably more mellow) municipal union workers and professional embalmers, as well as a group of forty-six unemployed blind men who were assumed to exhibit "little ambition, drive, or desire to compete" because of their lack of sight. The wife of one of the type A subjects told the cardiologists, "If you really want to know what's giving our husbands heart attacks, I'll tell you. It's stress, the stress they receive in their work, that's what's doing it."

The idea of a stressed but high-achieving subset of American society especially prone to heart disease captured the American imagination. In 1968, the surgeon Donald Effler wrote in *Scientific American*, "The heart attack is so common among professional people, executives, and men in public office that it has become almost a status symbol. If all the men in these groups who have had coronary attacks were forced to retire . . . , the shortage of manpower at the top levels of government, industry, and the professions in the U.S. would cripple the nation."

The type A link to heart disease has not stood up to modern investigation and is now generally considered an artifact of its time. More recent research has focused on the association of "negative affectivity" traits, such as depression, anxiety, and anger, with heart disease. The strongest evidence has emerged for depression, which seems to be an independent risk factor for coronary artery disease and increases the risk of poor outcomes, including death, after a heart attack. How does depression affect heart health? Possible mechanisms include elevating blood pressure, causing vascular inflammation, disturbing autonomic nervous system function, and increasing blood clotting. Also probably playing a role are unhealthy behaviors associated with depression, such as physical inactivity, smoking, and failure to take medications or adhere to medical advice.

Today a massive amount of epidemiological data associates heart disease with chronic emotional disorder—or disruption of the metaphorical heart. For example, individuals in unhappy marriages are at a much higher risk for heart disease than those in more joyous unions. The risk of myocardial infarction and death increases dramatically in the year following a broken romance.

These associations hold true even for animals we would not consider needing social connection. For example, in a study in the journal *Science*, researchers fed caged rabbits a high-cholesterol diet to study its effect on heart disease. Surprisingly, they found that animals in high cages got much more cardiovascular disease than ones in cages near the floor. The scientists investigated air circulation and other possible factors, without success. Then they discovered that the technician who delivered food played more often with the animals in the lower cages than with the ones near the ceiling. So they repeated the study, randomly dividing the rabbits into two groups: one group that was removed from their cages and petted, held, talked to, and played with, and another that remained in their cages and was ignored. The first group had 60 percent less aortic atherosclerotic surface area on autopsy than the second, despite having comparable cholesterol levels, heart rate, and blood pressure.

Socially stressed laboratory monkeys also develop more heart disease than matched controls. In another study in *Science*, male monkeys that had stranger monkeys introduced into their cages, often in the presence of an estrogen-laden female monkey, resulting in fights for dominance and less social huddling, developed more coronary artery disease than a control group of monkeys that was not stressed, even though cholesterol levels, blood pressure, blood sugar, and body weight were similar between the two groups. "Psychosocial factors," the authors concluded, "thus may help explain the presence of coronary artery disease (occasionally severe) in people with low or normal serum [cholesterol] and normal values for the other 'traditional' risk factors."

We paid little attention to "psychosocial" factors during fellowship. The focus of our seminars was on pressure-volume loops, cardiac work cycles, resistance of fluid-filled pipes, and capacitance of fluid-filled chambers. We concentrated on clinical trial design, biological mechanisms, and understanding the heart as a machine. As with most academic training programs, the fact that there was an emotional world that could damage (or heal) this pump was largely ignored.

Ironically, the view that heart disease results from unfulfilled social or psychological needs was widely accepted in primitive societies. That is almost certainly how people thought about heart disease in rural Punjab in the 1950s. Doctors at the hospital where my grandfather was pronounced dead did not know about the damaging effects of cholesterol and hypertension (Framingham results had not yet been broadly disseminated). They would have explained my grandfather's heart attack as the result of a sudden emotional shock (as when your neighbors bring a dead cobra into your home while you are having lunch with your family), or the years of social and financial struggle he endured after the Partition of India, or the loss of social connectivity that resulted from the fracturing and large-scale displacement of communities that had lived together for centuries, and in a sense they would have been right. Stress-induced surges of adrenaline can cause a stable atherosclerotic plaque to fissure and rupture, forming a thrombosis that can acutely block the artery and stop blood flow, thus causing a heart attack. Starved for oxygen, tissue begins to die. Irreversible cellular injury occurs within twenty minutes. And then, frequently, death.

Medicine today conceptualizes the heart as a machine. With advances in technology, perhaps this was inevitable. Drugs and devices have been responsible for much of the improvement in cardiovascular mortality over the past fifty years.

However, this narrow focus on biological mechanisms has hurt patients. We have overused stents and pacemakers. We have moved away from the emotional heart to a narrow focus on the biomechanical pump. The American Heart Association still does not list emotional stress among the key modifiable risk factors for heart disease—perhaps in part because serum cholesterol is so much easier to reduce than emotional and social disruption. We need a better way, one that recognizes the power and importance of emotions that the heart—the metaphorical heart—was believed to house for millennia. Though we know today that the heart is not the repository of the affections, it nevertheless remains the physiological canvas upon which our emotions are most easily written.

8

Pipes

The tragedies of life are largely arterial.
> —Sir William Osler, *Diseases of the*
> *Circulatory System* (1908)

The morning call was from the emergency room. A young man—an intern, in fact, who had been on rounds—had been admitted with chest pains. Could I come to evaluate him?

Such calls about hospital staff were dispensed with some regularity, and they rarely amounted to anything serious. Nevertheless, I hurried downstairs. The ER that morning was its customary mix of drunks and drug addicts. Nurses were just coming in for their day shifts. Stretchers were arranged like latticework in the corridors. There were the usual pressured announcements overhead ("Linda, stat to the trauma bay . . . Linda"). When I found the intern, Zahid Talwar, he was sitting on the side of a gurney, legs dangling, looking bored. He was about thirty, a Pakistani man with a long face and a long white coat who straightened up respectfully when I arrived. I introduced myself and asked him about the chest pain. It had started after dinner the night before, lasting about ten minutes. He had slept comfortably, but the pain recurred while he was walking to the bus stop that morning, persisting almost an hour. It was a dense pressure in the center of his chest that even he, a psychiatry intern, knew should be checked out. So he had decided to leave rounds and go to the ER.

I wasn't too concerned. Zahid was young, and his blood tests and electrocardiogram were normal. He had none of the usual Framingham risk factors for heart disease, such as diabetes, hypertension, or a regular smoking habit. I suspected he was suffering from acute pericarditis, a usually benign inflammation of the membrane around the heart often treated with over-the-counter anti-inflammatory drugs. Characteristic of pericarditis, the pain worsened when he took a deep breath. I told Zahid that if blood tests in six hours were normal, we would send him home. I joked there were easier ways to get out of internship duty.

Later that morning, I got a call from an ER physician informing me that Zahid's pain had resolved completely after he took ibuprofen, further confirming the diagnosis of pericarditis. For a moment I considered sending him home right then, but I decided to wait until the next set of blood tests was complete.

Just before leaving the hospital that evening, I ran into a physician assistant who told me that Zahid's subsequent blood tests showed abnormal enzyme levels, evidence of minor cardiac muscle damage. This took me by surprise. Pericarditis usually does not result in cardiac damage. I explained that the problem was probably *myo*pericarditis, in which inflammation of the surrounding membrane can partially involve the heart muscle. This, too, was relatively benign. The physician assistant asked me whether the young doctor should have a cardiac catheterization to rule out coronary blockages. I assured him that a thirty-year-old with no coronary risk factors did not have coronary artery disease. I instructed him to draw more blood, and to order an echocardiogram and call me at home if there were problems.

Zahid had chest pains through the night. Doctors who were called to see him attributed them to myopericarditis, the diagnosis written in the chart. At 2:00 a.m., he asked for more ibuprofen. "I told them, if it's pericarditis, give me more medication," he told me later. "Means, do whatever it takes to make the pain go away."

When I saw him in the morning, the pain had subsided. However, further blood tests showed evidence of continuing heart muscle injury, and an EKG now showed new, though nonspecific, abnormalities. Though I still doubted that he had coronary artery disease, I sent him to the cardiac catheterization lab for an angiogram.

I received a call about an hour later asking me to come over to the lab. When I arrived, the angiogram was playing on a computer screen. It showed a complete blockage of the left anterior descending (LAD) artery. The artery looked like a lobster tail, unnaturally terminating after several centimeters. X-rays showed severe dysfunction of the entire anterior portion of Zahid's left ventricle. My young patient—a *doctor*—had been having a heart attack for more than twenty-four hours.

●

If, as Osler said, the tragedies of life are mostly arterial, then the source of most of mankind's misery is the fatty plaque. By cutting off blood flow, obstructive arterial plaque is responsible for heart attacks and strokes, the most common ways we die. By the 1960s, the mechanisms underlying this process were being aggressively investigated. In 1961, the Framingham study confirmed that cholesterol is a risk factor for coronary heart disease, but it did not explain why. In the decade following, scientists showed that when the concentration of blood cholesterol gets too high, small cholesterol particles can burrow through the inner lining of blood vessels and take up residence inside the wall. This begins benign, but the cholesterol soon reacts with oxygen to form free radicals that injure nearby cells. As these injured cells release chemical signals— calls for help— white blood cells swarm to the site of injury. There, they transform into cells called macrophages that feed on the oxidized cholesterol. Bloated by this indigestible cholesterol, the macro-phages turn into "foam" cells, padding the vessel's wall. They continue to gobble up cholesterol until they pass the brink of rupture, vomiting a gooey paste into the wall. The domino effect continues as more macrophages are recruited to the site, multi-plying, causing the lesion to enlarge. Scar tissue is deposited to form a crust over what is now a malignant soup of fat, diges-tive enzymes, swarming macrophages, and dead cells—a full-fledged atherosclerotic plaque. In the beginning, the artery expands to compensate for the intrusion of plaque into the space within, but as the lesion gets bigger, the plaque eventually pushes into the vessel, hindering blood flow.*

The physiology of atherosclerotic plaque was mostly under-stood by the early 1960s, but how to treat it? As with any pipe, the first step is to pinpoint the blockage, not an easy feat in the dark caverns of the human body. On a temperate October day in 1958 in Cleveland, Ohio—just two years after Werner Forssmann received the Nobel Prize—Mason Sones, director of the cardiac catheterization lab at the Cleveland Clinic, came up with a solution to this problem.

Like Forssmann, Sones was a bit of a lunatic. Even in an era when doctors lived and breathed medicine, Sones topped the charts. He routinely worked until midnight, holding his ciga-rettes with sterile forceps while he smoked in the cath lab. Then, instead of going home to his wife and children, he'd peel off his stained white undershirt and go out for drinks at a nearby hotel. Nurses and secretaries were known to hide from him in the ladies' bathroom. He'd soon catch on, pounding on the door

---

*Obstructive plaque can stimulate "collateral circulation," or the formation of new blood vessels. Oxygen-deprived cells downstream from the obstruction re-lease chemical growth factors that signal primitive vascular cells to invade the hypoxic tissue, assembling into a plexus of new hollow tubes that link up into a complex network. This process, called angiogenesis, ensures that blood vessels permeate every region of the body. These new blood vessels—the heart's attempt to repair itself—limit the damage caused by a heart attack.

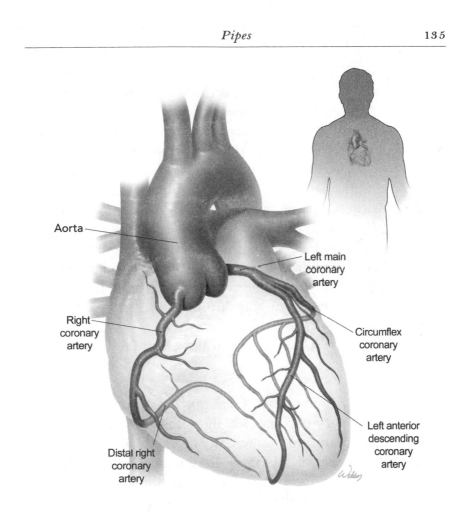

Coronary arteries (Courtesy of Scott Weldon)

whenever he had a task that demanded their immediate attention. Like Forssmann, Sones was brash and bullying. Like his great predecessor, he skipped animal studies and went straight to human demonstration. And like the German, he had the brazenness—and perhaps the good fortune—to go first.

The coronary arteries take off from the aorta, the main artery in the body, just beyond the aortic valve. In the 1950s, cardiologists, fearful of putting a catheter directly into the coronaries, would inject massive amounts of dye into the aortic root, hoping some of it would trickle into the coronaries so they could be visualized by X-ray. Such "nonselective" injection was a feint, a sort of foreplay, and it provided few useful images.

One October morning, Sones was getting ready to inject dye into the aortic root of a twenty-six-year-old man to image the vessel in preparation for open-heart surgery when, as he was moving the catheter into position, it slipped into the opening of the right coronary. I learned during my fellowship that because of the shape of the aortic arch, it is almost easier to insert a catheter into the right coronary than to avoid it. Sones knew this, too, and whenever the catheter slipped into the orifice, he would withdraw it a few millimeters to disengage it. However, this time, before he could do anything, his assistant stepped on the dye pedal and dumped 50 cc of dye into the artery.

In a letter to a colleague, Sones recounted the fateful episode:

> When the injection began I was horrified to see the right coronary artery become heavily opacified and realized that the catheter tip was actually inside the orifice . . . I ran around the table looking for a scalpel to open [the patient's] chest in order to defibrillate him by direct application of the paddles . . . Fortunately he was still conscious and responded to my demand that he cough repeatedly. After three or four explosive coughs his heart began to beat again.

He later wrote,

> Initially, I could feel only unbelievable relief and gratitude that we had been fortunate enough to avert a grievous disaster. [But] during the ensuing days I began to think that this accident might point the way for the development of a technique, which was exactly what we had been seeking.

Sones's technique, called coronary angiography, outlined the flow of blood in the coronaries using dye and X-rays, thus pinpointing the location of plaque. "I knew that night that we finally had a tool that would define the anatomic nature of coronary artery disease," he said. However, as is often true in medicine, diagnosis was only the first step toward a cure. It took almost two decades after Sones's breakthrough to develop this "cure."

In the meantime, scientists focused on perfecting nonsurgical treatments for patients who'd suffered heart attacks. In 1961, Desmond Julian, a cardiology fellow at the Royal Infirmary in Edinburgh, Scotland, published the first paper on the benefits of housing heart attack patients in a special cardiac care unit. "Many cases of cardiac arrest associated with acute myocardial ischemia could be treated successfully if . . . the cardiac rhythm of patients with acute myocardial infarction were monitored by an electrocardiogram linked to an alarm system," Julian wrote. Before the advent of such monitoring, most patients who suffered heart attacks were housed for weeks in rooms off the main medical ward, far from ringing phones and the hustle and bustle of the nurses' station, to give their hearts peace and quiet and a chance to heal. This benign neglect exacted a heavy toll, however. Senior cardiologists from that era have told me that when they would come to the medical wards early in the morning to draw blood, they'd often find one or two cardiac patients who had died quietly during the night.

Like other CCUs, Bellevue's had a bank of EKG monitors that continuously tracked patients' heart rhythms. Defibrillators and other resuscitation equipment were on standby. The nurse-to-patient ratio was 1:3 or sometimes even 1:2. Such vigilance saved lives. One morning, soon after my fellowship began, a middle-aged woman in her third day after a heart attack went into ventricular fibrillation, the chaotic rhythm that killed both my grandfathers. She had been feeling well and was eager to go home; her only complaint was of the EKG stickers irritating her skin. Then she slumped over. Her eyes rolled up in her head, and her face turned bluish, like an old bruise. If I had opened her chest at that point and held her fibrillating heart in my hand, it would have felt like a bag of swarming worms. I stepped into the hallway and shouted for an external defibrillator. An attending physician ran in and delivered two hard punches to her chest, "precordial thumps" that can sometimes terminate fibrillation, though that morning they did not. We inserted a board under the patient's body and started chest compressions. When the defibrillator was brought in, I applied the metal paddles to her bony frame. One 360-joule shock was all it took. She coughed twice, her pulse reappeared, and she took a deep breath. Her eyes opened wide, and she turned her head to face us, looking sheepish, puzzled by all the commotion. She had no idea we had saved her from certain death. Her roommate in fact was more traumatized. Rocking back and forth in her bed, she quietly asked me to draw the curtain closed.

•

So, by the early 1960s, cardiologists could image a coronary obstruction. But how to fix it? Surgeons were already bypassing vascular obstructions in the legs and in the heart using vein grafts harvested from various sites in the body. However, mortality and morbidity rates in these bypass operations were unacceptably high. So a cadre of zealots began to try to figure out ways to create new channels of blood flow, not around a blocked artery but through it.

One of these doctors was Charles Dotter, a radiologist at the University of Oregon. At a conference in Prague in 1963, Dotter predicted that the angiographic catheter could be "more than a tool for diagnostic observation. Used with imagination, it can become an important surgical instrument." Dotter—"Crazy Charlie," to some—was an odd bird: a mountain climber, ornithologist, and amphetamine addict. He fashioned guide wires for his procedures out of guitar string, and at conferences he blowtorched catheters out of Teflon tubing at his hotel. Once, in the middle of delivering a lecture on cardiac catheterization, he rolled up his shirtsleeve to reveal to the audience that he had placed a catheter in his own heart that morning. Then, as he continued to lecture, he connected himself to an oscilloscope to record the pressures from his cardiac chambers.

Dotter performed the first therapeutic procedure with a catheter, which he called angioplasty, on January 16, 1964, when an eighty-two-year-old patient named Laura Shaw, who had a blocked artery in her leg that had resulted in gangrene, was brought to his radiology lab. Her limb was crusty, dusky, and infected. Even though she was in terrible pain, she refused amputation. As a palliative measure, Dotter inserted a wire through the skin on the back of her knee and into the blocked artery and then sequentially passed concentrically enlarging plastic catheters over the wire to dilate the vessel, relieving the obstruction by packing the plaque onto the vessel wall "like footprints in the sand." The procedure was successful. Shaw's pain subsided, and the infection resolved. She succumbed two years later to a heart attack.

For this and subsequent leg procedures, Dotter received widespread publicity. In August 1964, *Life*, the most widely circulated periodical in the country, published a photo spread of Dotter posing oddball during one of his clog-clearing procedures. "Things have been both rewarding and at times frustrating," Dotter told the magazine. "In the early days of . . . angioplasty I had to accept a lot of unpleasant backbiting, such as 'He's a nut, you can't trust his uncontrolled, poorly documented case experience,' and worse. I'm glad I was thick-skinned enough to stick with it."

Angioplasty was simply unclogging a pipe, and in fact Dotter frequently referred to himself as a plumber. "If a plumber can do it to pipes, we can do it to blood vessels," he said. But his technique was coarse and crude, often resulting in a sort of snowplowing of plaque down the artery, where it could filter into smaller branches, obstructing them. Vessel injury was common, resulting in tears, bleeding, and scarring. Sometimes the plaque would dislodge and travel down the artery, causing infarction and tissue death. Though Dotter suggested that a more controlled dilation would be safer and more effective, he was never able to develop this method.

That critical step was left up to another German physician, Andreas Gruentzig, who began toying with Dotter's catheters in the late 1960s. Like so many of the great cardiac innovators, Gruentzig was an engineer at heart. His two-bedroom flat in Zurich was across the street from where James Joyce wrote much of *Ulysses*, and his kitchen table, laid out with drawings, knives, plastic tubing, air compressors, and epoxy glue, was in fact a portrait of an artist's work space. Gruentzig often worked all night fashioning prototype catheters. When colleagues would visit—at all hours, to the chagrin of Gruentzig's long-suffering wife—he would lead them to his kitchen and put them to work. With a mane of black hair and a burly mustache, Gruentzig was handsome and charismatic. Like Forssmann, his legendary predecessor, he was a risk taker, winging his single-engine plane low over the Swiss Alps on weekend getaways. But unlike Forssmann, he worked systematically and inspired followers.

Gruentzig set as his task adding an inflatable balloon to the end of his catheters that was thin but strong enough not to compress or burst when encountering arterial walls studded with plaque. He first tested these balloon catheters on anesthetized dogs that he smuggled into the hospital on gurneys under drapes. The dogs' arteries were stitched half closed to mimic an atherosclerotic blockage. When those experiments proved successful, Gruentzig went to work on human cadavers. On February 12, 1974, ten years after Dotter's first angioplasty, Gruentzig used one of his catheters to perform the first human balloon angioplasty on a sixty-seven-year-old patient with a severe stricture of the iliac artery, a major vessel in the leg. After the balloon was inflated, relieving the blockage, an ultrasound showed free-flowing circulation, and the patient's incapacitating leg pain vanished. Following this triumph, Gruentzig began to perform balloon angioplasty on a regular basis, handcrafting catheters for every new patient and meticulously tracking his results to deny voice to his critics. It was difficult, painstaking work. "If I had an enemy, I would teach him angioplasty," he wearily told a colleague.

However, the ultimate goal for Gruentzig and others was the coronary artery, whose disease was responsible for so much death around the world. "The legs were only my testing ground," Gruentzig said. "From the beginning I had the heart in mind." Dotter himself wrote that the development of coronary angioplasty was "one of radiology's most pressing responsibilities." However, the idea of balloon coronary angioplasty was heretical in the extreme. There were so many potential pitfalls. The balloon could puncture the artery, causing rapid hemorrhage and pericardial tamponade. The vessel could recoil and close, causing a massive heart attack. The heart could develop fibrillation and stop beating altogether. For years, Gruentzig's ideas were met with disdain, motivated by fear and perhaps not a small amount of jealousy. But he was a man of conviction, and there was nothing Gruentzig believed in more than himself.

Gruentzig meticulously pursued his vision. He forged collaborations on steerable catheters with American manufacturers, including the company that would eventually become the multibillion-dollar conglomerate Boston Scientific. He practiced on the coronary arteries of cadavers, then later on living patients undergoing bypass surgery, but only in vessels that were already bypassed or about to be bypassed, or were small and inconsequential. Gruentzig presented his results at cardiology meetings but, like Werner Forssmann, encountered skepticism and derision. Nevertheless, he bided his time, waiting for the right opportunity to present itself, a living person on whom to demonstrate his technique.

He finally got his chance on September 16, 1977, when

Adolph Bachmann, a thirty-seven-year-old insurance salesman, was transferred to the University Hospital in Zurich with chest pains. A coronary angiogram revealed a short obstructive plaque in the beginning portion of the left anterior descending artery. An emergency coronary bypass operation was scheduled for the following day, but Gruentzig persuaded Bachmann, who was afraid of open-heart surgery, and his doctors to allow him to perform balloon coronary angioplasty instead. The following morning, as a dozen cardiologists, surgeons, anesthesiologists, and radiologists looked on, Gruentzig threaded one of his balloon-tipped catheters into Bachmann's femoral artery, up his aorta, and into the opening of his LAD. Two out of Gruentzig's three balloons burst during preparations, but the third one remained intact. Two quick balloon inflations inside the coronary artery and blood began to flow normally down the vessel. The surgeons in the audience stared in disbelief. Gruentzig had restored blood flow to heart muscle without scalpel, saw, or heart-lung machine. It seemed impossible. Gruentzig was prepared to inject the LAD with Bachmann's own blood to wash away any dislodged plaque, but he did not have to. Bachmann's chest pains immediately subsided. A post-procedure angiogram showed almost complete resolution of the obstruction. (Ten years later, the artery remained open.) The only complication was a transient EKG abnormality that cleared up spontaneously.

At the American Heart Association conference in Miami that year, Gruentzig presented the results of his first four coronary angioplasties. True to his iconoclastic form, he presented his data (to raucous applause) wearing sandals. Afterward, Mason Sones, teary-eyed and by then battling lung cancer, told a colleague, "It's a dream come true."*

After years of working in obscurity, Gruentzig quickly be-

---

*A few years later, Sones said that the era of angioplasty was "the best time in medical history to have been alive, and I am deeply grateful for the privilege."

came one of the most famous cardiologists in the world. In 1980, three years after the first coronary angioplasty, he moved his research enterprise to Emory University in Atlanta, Georgia. Over the next five years, he helped to popularize angioplasty in the United States by performing approximately twenty-five hundred procedures. He had so much faith in his technique that he once had a cardiology fellow perform a coronary angiogram on Gruentzig himself. Gruentzig climbed onto the cath table at 5:00 p.m., underwent the procedure, and then went to pick up his wife, arriving at the department's Christmas party by 7:00. Incidentally, his coronary arteries were normal.

Gruentzig's procedure ushered in the field of interventional cardiology. In 1980, Marcus DeWood and colleagues used coronary angiography to show that patients suffering heart attacks have arterial clots that obstruct coronary blood flow. This discovery quickly led to the development of clot-busting drugs and the refinement of angioplasty procedures for the treatment of acute myocardial infarction. In 2001, when I began my fellowship, coronary angioplasty was already a sprawling business. One evening, wearing bloodstained scrubs, I ran into Bert Fuller, the kindly chairman at Bellevue. He was sporting his usual maroon sweater and pants that were at least a size too small. We walked together, chatting about my cath lab experiences. Outside Bellevue, it had snowed, and the sidewalk was slushy. "How little we knew," Fuller said, shaking his head as we waited in line in front of a truck to buy a cup of coffee. "When we started, cardiac catheterization was used only for unremitting chest pains. Now it has become routine."

Today several million angioplasties are performed worldwide every year, one million in the United States alone. In 1994, the Food and Drug Administration (FDA) approved the release of coronary stents, tiny metallic coils that are used in the clear majority of angioplasties today to keep ballooned arteries open. In the early years of the twenty-first century, stents began to be coated with chemicals that prevent scar tissue from forming. The first drug that was used was rapamycin, an antibiotic discovered in a soil mold on Easter Island that stops cell division. Nowadays, most stents used in the United States are coated with rapamycin or a similar drug, which has nearly eliminated in-stent scarring.

From a self-surgery in a tiny operating room in Eberswalde, Germany, cardiac catheterization has been transformed into a hugely profitable, multibillion-dollar industry. Unfortunately, Gruentzig never got a chance to witness this revolution. He and his second wife, a medical resident, died on October 27, 1985, when the private plane he was piloting crashed in a storm in rural Georgia. He was forty-six years old. That year was a tragic one for interventional cardiology. Smoking caught up with the field's heroes. Mason Sones died of metastatic lung cancer; Charles Dotter, ironically, of complications of coronary bypass surgery.

9

Wires

And pale and wan, and of all strength bereft,

. . .

My heart, as with an earthquake, then is cleft,
Which makes my pulse leave all its life behind.
                    —Dante Alighieri, from Sonnet IX

The old man shuffled slowly into my clinic room. He took off
his hat and collapsed into a cracking vinyl chair. I had seen
him before, last about two weeks ago. He had never looked
this bad.

He leaned forward, a bearded, wispy-thin gentleman in a
vintage suit whose bowler and neckerchief lent him an arcane,
vaudevillian air. "The shortness of breath is getting worse," he
growled in a raspy voice, not unlike Bob Dylan's. "The medications you prescribed aren't helping."

Jack, as he was called, had been a beneficiary of the pioneering heart surgeries of Walt Lillehei and others in the 1950s. A
diseased valve was surgically repaired when he was a child. With
no heart-lung machine, the surgeon used his little finger,
wedged into the wall of the right ventricle, to free up the mo
tion of the congenitally rigid valve.

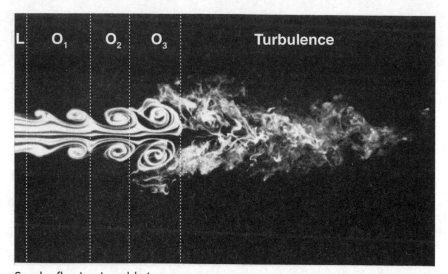

Smoke flowing in cold air (From James N. Weiss et al., "Chaos and the Transition to Ventricular Fibrillation," *Circulation* 99 [1999]. Reproduced by permission)

The procedure was successful, but over the years the valve leaked, eventually causing Jack's heart to weaken and enlarge like a worn-out balloon. Now his heart was pumping much less efficiently than normal, about 30 percent of full strength. He was getting winded after only a few steps. Several weeks prior, he'd collapsed on the stairs leading to his third-floor walk-up and had to be carried up by neighbors.

Gripping my hands like a banister, Jack hobbled onto the exam table. I put the rubber buds of the stethoscope in my ears. His waterlogged lungs crackled like Rice Krispies in milk. With my fingertips, I made tiny craters in his edematous legs. I asked him to take off his shirt so I could listen to his heart. Then I noticed it, rolled up in a yellow vest, strapped to his chest like some sort of talisman. "What is this?" I asked.

He took it off and handed it to me. "My magnet," he replied. It was wrapped in duct tape and must have weighed three or four pounds. I waved it at a cart sitting next to my desk. My arm wavered and then jerked gently as the magnet stuck to the metal.

"It's heavy," I said. He nodded. "Why do you have it?" I asked.

Magnetic fields dilate blood vessels, he explained. (I didn't know.) In fact, they have a host of salutary effects on the body, he told me.

He had first heard about magnets a few years back on short-wave radio; he had been using them ever since to relieve head-aches, heal minor cuts, and now support his failing heart. He even wore a magnetic belt—made with tiny domino magnets that he purchased from Radio Shack—to treat an abdominal hernia, which had gotten smaller. "Could it just be the pressure of the belt?" I asked.

"A plain belt didn't work," he replied.

He told me that ever since he started putting the magnet on his chest, his heart failure had improved. I reminded him that when we first met in the Bellevue Emergency Room a few months earlier, he was near death, literally drowning from the congestion in his lungs. "Just imagine where I would have been without the magnet," he said.

I had heard of magnets being used to treat chronic pain—even here the evidence was sketchy—but never to treat advanced heart failure. I wasn't sure what to say. "You should have told me," I said finally.

"You never asked," he replied.

He went on to say that I had given off a negative vibe when-ever the subject of alternative medicine had come up. Remem-ber when he had asked about milk thistle and taurine? (I didn't.) Apparently, I had been dismissive, almost scornful. He had asked me to call Gary Null, one of his "natural healers," to review his treatment protocol, but I never did. He had even consid-ered switching doctors because I had seemed "too dogmatic."

Heat rose to my face. Too dogmatic? Me? I remembered the book he had lent me, *The Clinician's Handbook of Natural Healing*, which lay on my coffee table, unopened. Now I wished I had looked at it, if only to show him what an open-minded doctor I was.

"I'm not aware of any good evidence for alternative therapies for heart failure," I stammered.

How did I know this without reading up on the current research? he demanded. I felt like a first-year fellow again, unprepared to argue my point. It didn't matter to Jack that I was the doctor or that I had made it through most of a cardiology fellowship or that I was, in fact, planning on specializing in the treatment of congestive heart failure. Like me, he wanted evidence. He was using my own paradigm against me.

Chastened by his criticism, I offered an apology, which he accepted. Then he told me that besides milk thistle and taurine, he had been taking more than a dozen other unproven off-the-shelf supplements: carnitine, glutathione, goldenseal, corn silk, dandelion, black cohosh, dimethylglycine, coenzyme Q, thiamine, alpha-lipoic acid, stinging nettles, oil of oregano, echinacea, magnesium, selenium, and copper. None were recorded in the chart.

Once the genie was out, he could hardly hold back. He removed the soles of his shoes, embedded with tiny neodymium magnets that he had purchased for forty-five cents apiece at a thrift store. He handed me his glasses; two round magnets were attached to the frames. (That's what those were!) A few years back, he said, he had had a serious lung infection, requiring treatment with several antibiotics for almost a year. He wasn't using magnets at the time. He was never going to make that mistake again.

Could it just be random, I asked, this association between magnets and health? Knowing that Jack was well versed in philosophy, I brought up Karl Popper's theory of science and the requirement of falsifiability. Suggest an ailment we can test, I said excitedly. We could conduct a small trial, on and off magnet therapy. He shrugged, unfazed. "I try to keep myself from analyzing it too much or talking myself out of the placebo effect," he said.

When he got up to leave, he handed me a tiny magnet as a

gift. "Keep it away from your wallet," he advised. "It'll erase your MetroCard."

•

It was on Wednesdays that Jack would come to see me at the Bellevue cardiology clinic. Like many of my patients, he was a clinic veteran who had been through several cycles of fellows. "I know I'm getting older when the doctors are getting younger," he quipped. The clinic was always packed. You'd get ten or twelve minutes per visit, max. You listened to the heart and lungs, went through the problem list, wrote a progress note, maybe wrote a prescription, and then it was off to see the next patient. No surprise, then, that Jack—and many other patients, I suspected—had adopted alternative medicine. I figured Dr. Null spent more time with Jack, listened to him, and showed that he cared. But did his natural remedies work? I took it as a challenge to prove to Jack that my way, informed by science, was better.

At a clinic visit a few weeks after Jack showed me his magnets, I spoke with him about his treatment options. "You have a weak heart," I said, slowly moving my outstretched fingers, as if palming a basketball, to illustrate. I brought up the option of an implantable defibrillator. The beeper-sized device would be inserted in Jack's chest to monitor his heartbeat and apply an electrical shock if the rhythm degenerated into something dangerous. It was like the paddles in the ER, but it would always be inside him. A special "biventricular" defibrillator would help to coordinate the contractions of Jack's failing heart. It might relieve his breathlessness and decrease the frequency of hospitalizations. It might even prolong his life.

Biventricular defibrillators then cost about $10,000 each. In the United States, where more than six million patients have heart failure and half a million new cases are diagnosed each year, if even a small fraction of patients like Jack received the device, the costs could reach billions. But apart from the money, a bigger question in my mind was whether the device was even right for Jack. He was probably going to live at least a year, but certainly no more than five. How did he want to die when his time came? Patients with heart failure mostly die in two ways: either by a sudden, "lights out" arrhythmia, in which the heart abruptly stops, or by progressive pump failure, in which the heart weakens to the point that it cannot deliver adequate blood and oxygen to the tissues. Pump failure is a horrible way to die. The symptoms it creates—nausea, fatigue, and unremitting shortness of breath—are some of the most torturous and feared in the human experience. Wasn't a sudden arrhythmia a better way for Jack to go than struggling for breath as his lungs filled with fluid from congestive heart failure? Sure, a defibrillator would prevent sudden death. But it would also take away the sudden-death *option*, potentially directing the dying process down painful, winding paths. Of course, when Jack's condition inevitably spiraled downward, he could always deactivate the device and prevent it from delivering a painful shock. However, in my experience, few patients ever did. Doctors rarely informed them of this option, and families, struggling to cope with the impending death of a loved one, were often reluctant to make that choice.

I did not go into these details with Jack, however. It was hard enough to fit any sort of discussion, let alone a drawn-out, morbid one, into a ten-minute office visit. I recommended he get a defibrillator. I wasn't sure it was the right decision, but the device, I figured, would at least help him in the short run. But none of this mattered anyway, because Jack quickly waved off my recommendation. He didn't want a defibrillator. With time, he was convinced, his magnets were going to work.

•

The heart is fundamentally an electrical organ. Without electricity, there would be no heartbeat. Electrical impulses stimulate special proteins in heart cells, causing them to draw together, resulting in contraction of the entire organ. Derangements in the rhythm of these impulses impair the heart's ability to pump blood. By the early part of the twentieth century, this was understood, and the heart's wires had been mapped. For example, physiologists knew that nearly every one of the three billion heartbeats that occur during a typical human lifetime begins with the spontaneous activation of cells in a region high up in the right atrium called the sinoatrial node, the heart's natural pacemaker. Through the flow of charged ions, the voltage of these cells periodically arrives at a threshold; this happens about once a second in a normal person at rest. That induces an electrical wave—an action potential—that spreads through the atria and travels down specialized conductive tissue—wires, really—into the ventricles, stimulating heart cells along the way. (Think of the pulse generated when you jerk the end of a rope up and down.) Just before the wave enters the ventricles, it passes through a narrow, relatively inert disk of tissue called the atrioventricular node. Here, the electrical impulse slows to a crawl for about a fifth of a second, giving the atria time to finish squeezing and filling the ventricles with blood. The wave then passes into the ventricles through thick bundles of tissue that rapidly and finely split into conductive filaments that extend through the ventricles like the roots of a tree. In this way, an impulse originating in one part of the heart quickly conducts through the entire organ, causing the right and left ventricles to contract almost simultaneously, ejecting blood into the lungs and the main body, respectively.

After a cardiac cell is stimulated, it enters a "refractory" period in which the cell becomes essentially quiescent; no electrical stimulus, no matter how intense, will elicit another response. This is a protective mechanism, preventing cardiac tissue from being rapidly and repeatedly activated. If the heart beats too fast, circulation can cease and the person will die.

There are several other layers of protection that ensure the stability of the human heartbeat. For example, if the sinoatrial

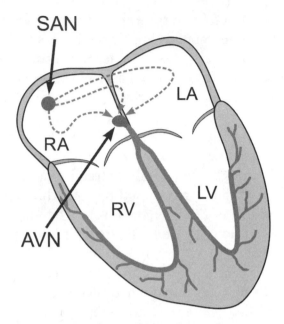

The heart's conduction system: SAN, sinoatrial node; AVN, atrioventricular node; RA, right atrium; LA, left atrium; RV, right ventricle; LV, left ventricle. Dashed lines represent atrial activation; solid lines represent pathways for ventricular activation. (Courtesy of R. E. Klabunde, www.cvphysiology.com, 2017)

node, the heart's natural pacemaker, becomes dysfunctional, any number of backup pacesetters in the heart can take over. These regions normally have different electrical properties and activate more slowly than the sinoatrial node, so their activity is ordinarily suppressed (their cells are in a refractory state) when the sinoatrial node is firing normally. But if one of these regions speeds up because of damage or disease or adrenaline release, it can usurp the sinoatrial node's pacemaking function.

By the turn of the century, this paradigm had largely been laid out. Scientists understood that the heartbeat is powered by electricity generated in the right atrium and conducted southward, stimulating billions of electrically coupled cells along the way. What took longer to appreciate is that when the heart stops beating, that is usually because of electricity, too.

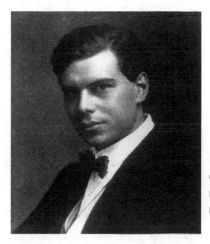

George Mines, circa 1914 (Courtesy of Physiological Laboratory, Cambridge University, England. Reprinted with permission)

The key figure to explain this connection was the Englishman George Mines, a product of the famed Cambridge School of Physiology. As a young man, Mines was a piano prodigy and briefly considered a career as a musician. This predilection for rhythms stayed with him. He received his PhD from Cambridge in 1912, when he was twenty-six. An avid photographer, Mines introduced the moving-image camera to cardiac physiology, recording the contractions of a pithed frog's heart by photographing it at fifteen frames per second on bromide paper, using a method pioneered by a close acquaintance, the cinematographer Lucien Bull. After he graduated from Cambridge, Mines did postdoctoral sabbaticals in England, Italy, and France before accepting a professorship in physiology at McGill University in Montreal. Mines's two most important discoveries—perhaps the most fundamental in the history of cardiac electrophysiology—were made during this period, in experiments he conducted on tortoises, fish, and frogs.

The first discovery was that small electrical channels can exist outside the normal conduction pathway in the heart. Normally, these extraneous circuits are excited uniformly and do not alter the heartbeat. But if one side of such a circuit—call it side A—has a longer refractory period than side B, because of

illness or electrolyte disturbance or injury from a heart attack, for example, it may be in a refractory state when a premature impulse arrives and will therefore not conduct. The
impulse will travel only down side B, which has recovered excitability because of its shorter refractory period. Mines's great
insight was that if side A *recovers excitability before the impulse
reaches the bottom of the circuit*, the impulse may conduct back
up side A and then again down side B (which quickly recovers
excitability because of its shorter refractory period), repeating
this pattern over and over. Theoretically, the impulse could
circulate indefinitely, without any further external stimulation.
With every rotation, a portion of the circulating wave can leak
out of the circuit and activate surrounding heart tissue, like a
lighthouse beacon sending its signal to faraway ships. In this
way, the circulating wave could usurp the activity of the sinoatrial node and become the dominant pacesetter in the heart.

    Mines called this phenomenon "reentry," and he was able
to visualize the circulating current in experiments on rings of
jellyfish. He published a classic figure still in use (akin to the
one shown below) that illustrates "circus movement" in these
myocardial circuits and how such movement can initiate rapid
arrhythmias. He also showed that cutting the circuit will in-

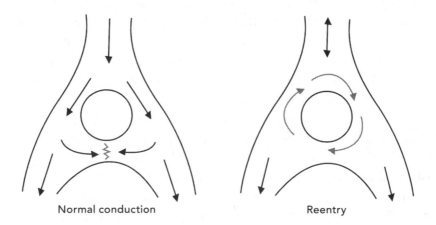

Normal conduction   Reentry

Cardiac reentry (Created by Liam Eisenberg, Koyo Designs)

stantly terminate the circulating wave, an observation that is the basis for surgical treatment of many arrhythmias today.

The modern depiction of reentry preserves Mines's essential insight. In this scheme, a circulating (or spiral) wave is set up in the presence of nonconductive tissue, such as a scar formed after a heart attack. If the scar is small compared with the wavelength of the impulse, the waves hardly notice it—as when water waves pass over a tiny pebble unperturbed.

But if the obstacle is large, the wave can break, the edges lagging behind as the rest of the wave moves ahead, thus causing the segments to begin to curl (as when flowing water encounters a large rock and forms an eddy current downstream). Far enough out, the wave edges become the center of circular (or spiral) waves.

The circular pattern reflects the need for refractory heart tissue to return to an excitable state in order for the wave to propagate and not die out. The simplest pattern to do this is a spiral, that iconic image of psychedelia, that anchors at one point, circulates, and slowly moves outward. As Mines discovered in his experiments on jellyfish, these spiral waves are self-sustaining: they can constantly reenter tissue that has recovered its excitability and persist indefinitely.

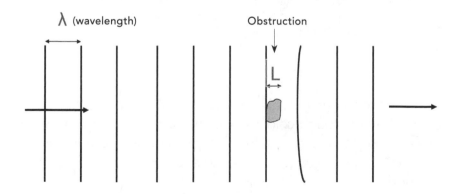

Wave hitting a small obstruction

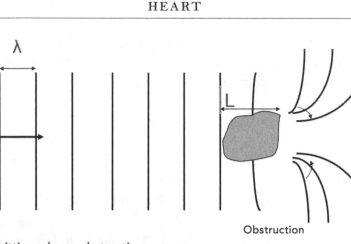

λ

L

Obstruction

Wave hitting a large obstruction

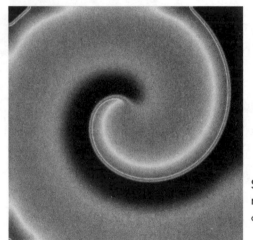

Spiral wave in a computer
model of cardiac tissue (Courtesy
of Alan Garfinkel)

Spiral waves are ubiquitous in nature. They are created when
smoke flows through cold air (see the picture on page 146) or
when water flows across pebbles. They occur in superconductors
and multicellular aggregates of amoebas, and in many chemical
reactions, too. Even the visible mass in the universe is organized
into spiral galaxies. With so many natural manifestations, it is
no surprise that this pattern is seen in the heart as well.

Though Mines observed reentry only in lower animals, mostly fish, the phenomenon was soon confirmed in human hearts in 1924. It is now widely accepted that spiral wave reentry underlies most abnormally fast heart rhythms, including ventricular fibrillation, the most common cause of cardiovascular death in the Western world.

In ventricular fibrillation, the heartbeat is so rapid and irregular that effective pumping of blood ceases to the brain, lungs, and other vital organs, resulting in a precipitous drop in blood pressure and the almost immediate onset of cell death. Though the heart is still quivering, blood flow has essentially stopped.* "Sudden cardiac failure does not usually take the form of a simple ventricular standstill," the Scottish physiologist John Alexander MacWilliam wrote in 1889. "It assumes, on the contrary, the form of violent, though irregular and uncoordinated, manifestations of ventricular energy." Every hour in the United States, forty people suffer an out-of-hospital cardiac arrest, mostly because of ventricular fibrillation. Fewer than one in ten survive. Ninety percent don't even make it to the hospital alive. Ethnic minorities and lower socioeconomic communities fare the worst, perhaps because of a lack of access to external defibrillators and a lack of education in bystander CPR. Survival after in-hospital cardiac arrest isn't much higher, about 25 percent. During the past several decades, mortality has decreased because of the proliferation of cardiac care units, community-based emergency rescue programs, and developments in cardiac electrophysiology. Yet ventricular fibrillation remains a death sentence for millions worldwide. An American dies of cardiovascular disease (including stroke and heart failure) every thirty-three seconds, accounting for about one in four deaths nationwide, and the terminal event in most of

---

*Ventricular fibrillation was probably first described by Andreas Vesalius, who observed that animals deprived of oxygen develop a wavy, wriggling motion of the heart.

those deaths is ventricular fibrillation. Purveyor of life, the heart is also its Grim Reaper.

Ventricular fibrillation most often occurs in diseased hearts, where damaged cells and disrupted electrical signaling create the conditions for reentry. However—and this should come as a shock—fibrillation can occur in *normal* hearts, too. In what was perhaps his most important discovery, Mines experimentally determined that there is a narrow period in the cardiac cycle—a "vulnerable period," he called it, about ten milliseconds in duration—during which a stimulus—an electrical shock or even a punch to the chest, in which mechanical energy is converted to electrical energy—can cause a perfectly normal heart to fibrillate and stop. To show this, Mines developed an apparatus to deliver single electrical shocks via taps of a Morse key to platinum electrodes placed on the ventricles of a rabbit's heart. In a number of instances, he found that "a single tap of the Morse key *if properly timed* would start fibrillation." The timing was crucial. "The stimulus employed would never cause fibrillation unless it was set in at a certain critical instant," Mines wrote. A stimulus delivered before the vulnerable period would do nothing; after the vulnerable period, the stimulus would merely initiate an extra heartbeat. But a stimulus applied within the vulnerable period could excite tissue just recovering from the last beat and precipitate fibrillation. In his 1913 report "On Dynamic Equilibrium in the Heart," Mines wrote that his findings "suggest an explanation of the important and interesting condition of *delirium cordis*," or madness of the heart.

The vulnerable period is crucial to understanding why normal hearts can self-electrocute. For example, when a healthy young athlete drops dead after getting a blow to the chest from a baseball or hockey puck, it is because the heart was hit during its vulnerable period. Scientists have confirmed the presence of the vulnerable period in mammals by slamming a baseball mounted at the end of an aluminum shaft into the chests of eight- to twelve-week-old anesthetized piglets at various times in the cardiac cycle. They found that when the impact occurs within a narrow window 10 milliseconds long and approximately 350 milliseconds after the previous heartbeat, it can induce cardiac arrest.

The explanation behind ventricular fibrillation in normal hearts is often also reentry. In a diseased heart with scar tissue, the mechanism is obvious: as we have seen, a wave breaks by interacting with inert scar tissue, forming spirals out of its edges. But reentry can occur even when there is no scar. In this case, a wave breaks by interacting with another wave, spinning around the refractory tissue formed in the other wave's wake as if a scar were present. This is known as "functional" reentry (as opposed to the "anatomic" reentry) and is just as deadly. The impulse that induces the spiral wave must occur at exactly the right time and place to collide with the wake of a previous wave. This is precisely the vulnerable period that Mines discovered in his rabbit experiments.

The first experimental observation of cardiac spiral waves was made by José Jalife and his colleagues at Syracuse University in 1992 and published in the journal *Nature*. Using a special camera to detect fluorescence from canine heart tissue injected with specific chemicals, they produced an image with the shape of a counter-rotating spiral with a size of about two centimeters. Jalife's group found that these spirals often anchor at scars or other inhomogeneities and can theoretically circulate indefinitely, each turn bringing the signal back to full strength, as Mines first showed.

Jalife also discovered that a spiral wave does not have to remain at a fixed position. When the spiral moves, it can start to meander, like a top slowing down on a table, its tip tracing a curlicue pattern. Eventually, the spiral wave can pick up so many oscillations that it breaks up, creating multiple independent spirals that stimulate the heart in a disordered fashion, as when waves collide at the shore, leaving thick, turbulent foam. This is ventricular fibrillation, an arrhythmia so fervent, so committed, so devoted to its mission that you literally have to shock it out of the heart to make it stop. The Scottish physiologist MacWilliam wrote of ventricular fibrillation in 1897, "The ventricular muscle is thrown into a state of irregular contraction, whilst there is a great fall in the arterial blood pressure. The ventricles become dilated with blood as the rapid quivering movement of their walls is insufficient to expel their contents." This is essentially electrical chaos, and the heart (and its owner) quickly die.*

In a 2000 study in the *Proceedings of the National Academy of Sciences*, Alan Garfinkel and his colleagues at UCLA imaged slices of pig hearts using a special microscope to show that when the tissue fibrillated, spiral waves were breaking up into multiple new waves that activated the heart in a chaotic pattern. It is not known precisely why spiral waves break up, resulting in fibrillation, but it is believed to depend on how quickly heart cells recover their ability to be re-excited, a property known as restitution. Restitution depends on many factors, but it can be amplified by lack of coronary blood flow—the mechanism that killed both my grandfathers—as well as by surges of adrenaline during psychological stress. Whatever the reason, when heart cells become more excitable, a spiral wave can become exquisitely sensitive to small perturbations in the electrical environment, picking up oscillations and setting up the conditions for breakup. "Steepening" of cardiac restitution may even be the mechanism behind "voodoo death," the mysterious, sudden demise documented by anthropologists that often occurs during periods of intense emotional stress, such as after a witch doctor's curse. Beta-blocking drugs that antagonize adrenaline have

---

*The idea that an excitable system can degenerate into chaos was first suggested by David Ruelle and Floris Takens in a 1971 paper titled "On the Nature of Turbulence." They proved mathematically that a system containing three or more coupled oscillations is inherently unstable. Their predictions were experimentally confirmed in studies of fluid dynamics and later electronic materials. Their work showed that ventricular fibrillation is a form of spatial and temporal chaos.

proved effective in preventing such fatal arrhythmias, which is perhaps why Mitch Shapiro, the Bellevue electrophysiologist, often said that beta-blockers should be put into New York City's water supply.

•

Mines's research on reentry and the vulnerable period inspired a new era in cardiac electrophysiology. Unfortunately, he did not live long enough to see the impact of his work. On the chilly Saturday evening of November 7, 1914, a janitor entered Mines's laboratory at McGill to find him lying unconscious under a lab bench with monitoring equipment attached to his body. He was rushed to the hospital but died shortly before midnight without recovering consciousness. Though an autopsy was inconclusive, medical historians believe his death was the result of experimentation on the vulnerable period in a human: himself. This speculation was fueled by a lecture that Mines delivered to McGill faculty one month before his death, when he was twenty-eight. In the talk, Mines spoke in praise of self-experimentation, referring to the work of contemporaries who severed their own nerves to understand the nature of skin sensations or swallowed a plastic tube to study the physiology of digestion. Evidently, Mines decided to put his theory of the vulnerable period to the test on himself. Mines did not know about Werner Forssmann. His tragic self-experiment predated the great German's self-catheterization by fifteen years.

10

Generator

When a condition is recognized as offering only a fatal or hopeless outlook, desperate measures seem less desperate and with application and courage not infrequently can be made safe.
—Charles P. Bailey, cardiac surgeon, Hahnemann Medical College, Philadelphia

"I told him that if he doesn't do something, he's going to be dead by the end of the year," Shawn, my magnet-wearing patient Jack's visiting nurse, told me on the phone one afternoon. "His heart is going to conk out, and he doesn't have time to play with these so-called nutraceuticals." Shawn paused, obviously frustrated. "You know what he said to me?" Shawn spit out the words in disgust. " 'Will it be painless?' "

I'd been calling Jack, my clinic patient, about once a week to check on him, but despite worsening heart failure he'd been resistant to my recommendations, convinced that his herbals and magnets would eventually work. Because of a lack of family and social support, Jack wasn't eligible for a heart transplant. There was no one available to assist him with chores or ensure he'd make it to his appointments or take his medicine. His only options were a $40,000 surgically implanted defibrillator—or hospice. I didn't hear anything for a few days. Then Shawn called to tell me that Jack was feeling sick again. He was sleeping sitting up in a chair because of the fluid accumulating in his lungs and was waking up every couple of hours gasping for air. Shawn had finally persuaded him to get the device.

I admitted Jack to the CCU at Bellevue and scheduled a cardiac catheterization prior to the implant. True to form, he quickly became annoyed with the hospital staff. One morning I was urgently paged to the unit because Jack was fighting with the nurses to go home. When I arrived, he was in a small, curtained space, lying on crumpled sheets in a fetal position. Thin plastic tubing delivering supplemental oxygen was pressed tightly against his sunken cheeks. I immediately turned the green knob controlling the flow of oxygen. A tiny ball bearing shot up in a plastic meter, suspended by the increased flow of air.

"I'm having pain in the middle of my chest," Jack said, without looking at me. A stained white knit cap had replaced his bowler. He looked even more emaciated than when I'd seen him in the clinic. I felt pity, but a bit angry, too. "This is why you need an angiogram, Jack," I said.

"You should have done it this morning," he growled, his eyes flashing anger even as they tried to close. "That's another day lost."

I told him the test was scheduled for the following day. If his coronaries were clean, we would implant the defibrillator immediately afterward.

"You're saying one thing; other people are saying something else."

"Well, I'm running the show here," I said quickly. As a senior cardiology fellow, it was nice to be able to say that I was finally in charge, at least of the care of my clinic patients.

"The consent form mentioned emergency bypass surgery," Jack continued monotone. "I don't want that."

That was just consent-form boilerplate, I explained. Every possible risk had to be included on the form in the unlikely event of a serious complication.

"My life was fine until you came in and started pushing your weight around," Jack said, trying to sit up.

"I think you're misinterpreting."

"It's my life!"

"Of course it is, Jack, but—"

"No!" he screamed pathetically. "I know what you're doing, trying to make some money off of me. Look, I'd rather die. Just let me die. I'm not afraid to die; I just want to go the right way."

I really did feel sorry for Jack. Obviously, the last thing he wanted to admit is that he needed me or modern cardiology to keep him alive. But there wasn't much more I could offer apart from the technology with which I had been trained. And though I still wasn't sure that a defibrillator was the right choice, once the decision was made, there was no point in ambivalence.

"I'm trying to help you, Jack," I said, sitting down. "I've done everything you've asked me to. I even reached out to Dr. Null"—the natural healer—"for his treatment protocol, but he wouldn't take my call. His assistant said he doesn't even know who you are."

(Null, I later learned, was a well-known alternative-health practitioner who denied that HIV causes AIDS, was opposed to vaccinations, and peddled dietary supplements he produced to treat various serious disorders, including cancer.)

"How is that my fault?" Jack barked.

"Look, Jack, I don't want to make you do something you don't want to do," I said, close to giving up. "I thought you wanted the device. If you didn't want it, you shouldn't have come to the hospital. You've wasted a lot of effort for nothing."

Outside the curtain there was rustling, probably an intern listening in. Jack straightened up. "I told you from the beginning that I thought you were too dogmatic," he said. "Unfortunately, your medications didn't work, and now we're back to where we started. I don't blame you; you're used to telling people what to do. But it isn't going to work with me."

But, in the end, it did work. After getting a shot of Ativan, Jack appeared soothed and agreed to proceed with the implant.

By then, I think he knew there were no other options available to him. But, pointing his finger at me in mock anger, he said, "If I hear you bragging that you finally got me, I'm going to get you."

•

In the decades after George Mines's trailblazing work in cardiac electrophysiology, electricity became widely available in industrialized countries. By the 1930s, 90 percent of urban residents in the United States had access to electrical power. From streetcars to lightbulbs to household appliances, electricity revolutionized the way people lived. Of course, by then scientists knew that electricity powered the heart, too. But when the heart's wiring failed, could *man-made* power be used to control the heart like any automatic dishwasher? This was a challenge that occupied a generation of researchers.

One of the first steps to meeting this test was taken by the cardiologist Paul Zoll at Beth Israel Deaconess Medical Center in Boston. During World War II, Zoll was assigned to an army hospital in England, where he served as the cardiologist on a surgical team. As he watched trauma surgeons remove shrapnel from soldiers' hearts, Zoll was struck by how excitable the heart muscle was. "You just touch it and it gives you a run of extra beats," he wrote. "So why should the heart that is so sensitive to any kind of manipulation die because there's nothing there to stimulate [it]?"

After the war, Zoll set out to treat patients with complete heart block, a common condition in which the heart's conduction system becomes diseased. In complete heart block, normal electrical impulses from the atria do not reach the ventricles. The ventricles, the main pumping chambers, must generate their own rhythm through a backup pacesetter that is usually much slower than the atria's. Patients with heart block often have a dangerously slow heartbeat. They are frequently short of breath and fatigued. They sometimes faint because of low blood flow. In rare cases, they may experience cardiac arrest and sudden death.

In his first experiments, Zoll slid an electrode down the esophagus of an anesthetized dog, positioning it a few centimeters from the left ventricle to maximize the electrical stimulus to the heart. To his amazement, he found that he could capture the heartbeat with an externally generated impulse. Zoll realized that in an emergency, there would be no time to pass an electrode into the mouth and down the food pipe of an unconscious patient, so in his next set of experiments, he dispensed with the esophageal electrode and applied electrodes directly to the chest. The chest electrodes worked, too; they just required a larger current to pass the electricity through the ribs and chest muscles. The timing of the external impulses had to be perfect, however; stimulating the heart during the vulnerable period could cause it to fibrillate. So Zoll created algorithms to properly trigger the stimulus from an EKG tracing.

External pacing worked in human volunteers, but it was torturously painful. The electric current would cause agonizing contractions of the chest muscles and quickly blister and ulcerate the skin. Moreover, like the rest of the hospital, external pacemakers were powered by the municipal electrical grid. Power cords had to be strung along hospital corridors and even down stairwells when patients wanted to ambulate. The grid was prone to shutdowns and failure, hardly reassuring when treating a pacemaker-dependent patient with complete heart block. External pacing was therefore only a short-term therapy for heart block.

For a more durable solution, a revolutionary idea emerged: to implant a pacemaker *inside* the body, allowing it to deliver a stimulus directly to the heart rather than to the chest muscles. The heart has few sensory nerve endings, so intracardiac pacing would not be painful. Moreover, powered by its own battery, an implantable pacemaker could be long-lasting and more reliable.

The concept of direct cardiac pacing materialized in a familiar place: the Department of Surgery at the University of Minnesota. Walt Lillehei, the pioneer of cross-circulation, was learning that conduction block was a frequent complication of his open-heart surgeries, either with cross-circulation or, after 1954, with the heart-lung machine. Suturing a ventricular septal defect could sever conduction pathways or cause enough tissue inflammation to disturb the pathways temporarily. During a morbidity and mortality conference at the university in 1956, a physiologist suggested that directly pacing the heart through an electrode on the heart's surface could rectify this problem. It would allow stimuli to be delivered to the heart at much lower voltage and be more dependable than external pacing of the chest wall.

Lillehei's team took this idea to the lab in Millard Hall. They created heart block in anesthetized dogs by passing a suture around the top portion of the ventricular conduction system. As expected, the dogs' heart rate quickly plummeted. They then stitched a wire into the outer wall of the heart, connected it to a pulse generator, and found that the heart rate picked right up.

After experiments with some fifty dogs, Lillehei used this "myocardial wire" for the first time in a human being on January 30, 1957. The six-year-old girl developed heart block during repair of a ventricular septal defect. With the wire in place and connected to a generator, the girl's ventricular rate increased immediately from thirty to eighty-five beats per minute, and she survived the operation. Lillehei was soon using the myocardial wire whenever a patient showed signs of heart block during or after open-heart surgery. His device was the first electrical instrument left inside the human body for any extended period, and it worked beautifully. However, it too was only a temporary fix because the wire had to be brought out of the chest through a surgical incision to be hooked up to a generator, thus creating a possible site of infection. It was designed to treat short-term, postsurgical heart block, albeit more effectively than external pacing.

Like much of what Lillehei did as a surgeon, there was no precedent for the myocardial wire. There was no way of knowing up front that it would work, that it wouldn't cause a host of complications—infection, bleeding, scarring—that putting a piece of metal inside the human body and leaving it there, tunneling a portion of it out through a break in the skin that could serve as a portal for germs, wasn't totally ridiculous. It was impossible to know any of this without trying. But Lillehei, more than any doctor of the twentieth century, specialized in trying the outlandish.

A long-term solution to complete heart block was needed, however. Older adults frequently develop chronic heart block because of myocardial infarction or age-related scarring and may require pacing for months, even years, to remain alive. Between 1957 and 1960, research groups from all over the world raced to design and test a fully implantable pacemaker. But in the end, Wilson Greatbatch, an unassuming electrical engineer at the University of Buffalo, was the first to succeed.

As with so many great cardiac innovations of the past century, the inspiration for Greatbatch's invention was a mistake. In the early 1950s, Greatbatch was working on a livestock farm near Ithaca, New York, testing instruments to monitor heart rate and brain waves in sheep and goats, when he learned about heart block from two surgeons doing a summer research sabbatical there. "When they described it, I knew I could fix it," Greatbatch later wrote. A few years later in Buffalo, Greatbatch was working with the newly invented transistor when he accidentally installed a resistor into a circuit he was testing, causing it to give off a signal that pulsed for 1.8 milliseconds, stopped for a second, and repeated—a rhythm that mimicked the human heartbeat. "I stared at the thing in disbelief and then realized this was exactly what was needed to drive a heart," Greatbatch wrote. "For the next five years, most of the world's pacemakers used [this circuit], just because I grabbed the wrong resistor."

In the spring of 1958, Greatbatch visited Dr. William Chardack, chief of surgery at the Veterans Affairs Hospital in

Buffalo, to explain his idea. Chardack was enthusiastic. "If you can do that, you can save ten thousand lives a year," he told Greatbatch. So Greatbatch went back to his workshop and fashioned a prototype device out of two Texas Instruments transistors. Three weeks later, Chardack implanted it into a dog. The two men watched in awe as the tiny device took over the heartbeat. "I seriously doubt if anything I ever do will give me the elation I felt that day when my own two-cubic-inch piece of electronic design controlled a living heart," Greatbatch wrote. From antiquity to modern times, philosophers and physicians had dreamed of taking charge of the human heartbeat. And finally it was possible, using simple circuit elements that were widely available. It was a seminal moment in the history of science.

However, Greatbatch's device had problems. It was sealed with electrical tape, so body fluids caused it to malfunction after a few hours. "The warm moist environment of the human body proved a far more hostile environment than outer space or the bottom of the sea," Greatbatch wrote. So he worked to cast the electronics in solid epoxy to make them more impervious, thus increasing their life span to four months. With no external funding, and splitting his time between Chardack's crowded lab and a small workshop in the barn behind his house, Greatbatch worked on the critical problems standing in the way of permanent cardiac pacing: battery life, proper insulation, and rising stimulation thresholds requiring higher and higher current to control the heart over time. (In the process, Greatbatch invented the first long-lasting lithium battery, still in use today.) By the late summer of 1959, Greatbatch had used up his personal savings of $2,000 to handcraft fifty implantable pacemakers. Forty were tested on animals; the remainder went into humans. The first human implant took place on April 7, 1960, in a seventy-seven-year-old man with complete heart block. He survived for eighteen months. The wires were hooked up to the outer wall of the ventricle, but later, using techniques developed by Wilfred Bigelow, the Canadian surgeon who pioneered surgical hypothermia, wires were passed through veins and directly into the heart. The Chardack-Greatbatch pacemaker worked remarkably well. One of the first patients to get one was electronically paced for more than twenty years and died in her eighties.

In the fall of 1960, Greatbatch and Chardack licensed their implantable pacemaker to a small Minneapolis company called Medtronic, which had been started by Earl Bakken, an electrical engineer who worked with Lillehei. Production began almost immediately. By the end of the year, the company had orders for fifty pacemakers at $375 apiece. Greatbatch continued to work on the device, testing transistors and other components in two ovens and a workbench set up in his bedroom in upstate New York. (The U.S. Minuteman nuclear missile program subsequently adopted many of Greatbatch's quality-control measures.) The demand for cardiac pacemakers quickly skyrocketed. Approximately 40,000 units were implanted in 1970 and about 150,000 in 1975. Today there are more than one million units in use around the world. In 1984, the National Society of Professional Engineers selected the implantable pacemaker as one of the ten most important engineering contributions to society over the preceding half century and honored Wilson Greatbatch, the humble engineer from upstate New York, as its inventor.

•

In addition to complete heart block, a deadly-slow arrhythmia, the other great problem cardiac electrophysiologists were grappling with at mid-century was ventricular fibrillation, the *fast* arrhythmia that was responsible for most sudden deaths across the world. At the turn of the century, Jean Louis Prévost and Frédéric Battelli, two researchers at the University of Geneva, discovered that electricity could be used not only to provoke ventricular fibrillation but to tame it as well. They were able to induce fibrillation in animals with relatively weak alternating current and then terminate it with a much larger "defibrillatory" jolt, resetting the heartbeat. Decades later, in 1947, the American surgeon Claude Beck successfully used electrical defibrillation for the first time in an operating room, on a fourteen-year-old boy at the Case Western Reserve University Hospital in Cleveland who went into cardiac arrest following a chest operation. The boy survived to be discharged from the hospital. Beck later wrote that defibrillation was a tool for saving "hearts too good to die." He envisioned the therapy as being "at the threshold of an enormous potential to save life."

As was the case with electronic pacing, externally applied defibrillation came first. In 1956, Harvard's Paul Zoll, who also pioneered external pacing, performed the first successful external defibrillation in a human subject. Other scientists, most notably William Kouwenhoven, a professor of electrical engineering at Johns Hopkins, also made seminal contributions. Kouwenhoven worked on external defibrillation for decades, mainly in rats and stray dogs. By 1957, he had assembled a defibrillator in his research lab on the eleventh floor of the Johns Hopkins Hospital. That March, a forty-two-year-old man arrived in the emergency room at two o'clock in the morning complaining of indigestion. He was actually having an acute myocardial infarction, and while undressing, he collapsed in ventricular fibrillation. The admitting resident, Gottlieb Friesinger, had heard about Kouwenhoven's defibrillator and raced upstairs to get it while an intern attempted to resuscitate the patient. Friesinger persuaded a security officer to let him into Kouwenhoven's lab, where he picked up the hefty device, nearly two hundred pounds, and wheeled it to the ER. With one electrode at the top of the breastbone and another just below the nipple, he delivered two shocks to revive the dying man. It was the world's first successful emergency defibrillation for cardiac arrest.

Kouwenhoven's research produced an unusual and unexpected side benefit. In experiments on dogs in the late 1950s, Guy Knickerbocker, a graduate student in Kouwenhoven's lab, noticed that blood pressure rose slightly when defibrillator paddles were pressed into position, even before any electrical current had been administered. Collaborating with James Jude, a surgeon, Knickerbocker showed that pressing on the chest can compress the heart and cause blood to temporarily circulate, thus increasing blood pressure. His observation set the stage for the introduction of chest compressions during cardiopulmonary resuscitation, the standard treatment used today. Within a year, this technique was being taught to firefighters and other rescue personnel. The discovery, serendipitously, benefited Knickerbocker personally. In 1963, his father underwent successful CPR during cardiac arrest after a heart attack.

External defibrillators quickly proliferated in the new cardiac care units of the 1960s. The machines were at the ready to treat the arrhythmic disturbances of heart disease, if not the disease itself. Monitoring in these units confirmed that ventricular fibrillation was the most common cause of cardiac arrest and sudden death. In 1961, a group led by Bernard Lown at Harvard incorporated a timer to synchronize the defibrillator with an EKG to avoid delivering shocks to the heart during the vulnerable period.

But as was the case with pacemakers, external defibrillators were unwieldy, and the shocks they delivered—in the rare cases when patients were still conscious—were painful. Moreover, they relied on bystander administration, hardly infallible during an emergency. Therefore, as with pacemakers, the goal became to miniaturize, automate, and implant them inside the body.

Though several groups were involved in the invention of external defibrillation, only one, led by Michel Mirowski at Sinai Hospital in Baltimore, was responsible for the creation of the implantable defibrillator. As a Jew born and raised in Warsaw, Mirowski led a peripatetic life. In 1939, as an adolescent, he left his family and fled his country after the German invasion and occupation of Poland. (He was the only member of his family to survive the war.) He ultimately returned to Poland. After the war, he did his medical training in France. A Zionist, he eventually moved to Israel. In 1966, when he was already a practicing cardiologist, he experienced a life-changing tragedy when his close friend and mentor, Harry Heller, died of ventricular tachycardia, a malignant rhythm that is often a precursor of ventricular fibrillation. Like so many traumatized by sudden cardiac death, it became his lifelong obsession.

In 1968, Mirowski moved to the United States. As chief of the new coronary care unit at Sinai Hospital, he negotiated time to pursue his own work in the basement of the hospital's research building. His project, conceived in Israel after Heller's death, was to build an implantable defibrillator. Mirowski paired up with Morton Mower, another cardiologist, and together they created a blueprint for the device. Mirowski knew that a strong electrical shock was needed to terminate ventricular fibrillation. However, he believed that with external defibrillation, most of this energy was wastefully dissipated in the tissues around the heart. He wondered whether the discharge of a simple capacitor, an electronic element that stores charge, might be sufficient to terminate fibrillation if the capacitor was in direct contact with the heart. Working with engineers, Mirowski and Mower designed circuitry to detect ventricular fibrillation and trigger the charging of a capacitor by a battery. The challenges were enormous: miniaturizing the circuits, constructing electronics to ensure the delivery of appropriate shocks (while avoiding inappropriate ones that could put healthy patients *into* ventricular fibrillation), and assembling a generator powerful enough to deliver multiple shocks for each fibrillation episode. The pair worked alone, like Greatbatch, and like Greatbatch they used their own money to pay for experimental animals and electrical components. At one point, they stole spoons from a nearby restaurant to make the implantable electrodes. Mirowski had great focus and will. His "three laws" were these: Don't give up. Don't give in. And beat the bastards.

In August 1969, Mirowski and Mower put a metal catheter

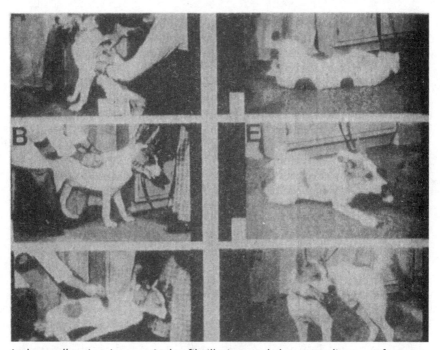

A dog collapsing in ventricular fibrillation and then standing up after successful defibrillation (Courtesy of *Pacing and Clinical Electrophysiology*)

inside a dog's superior vena cava and a metal plate—a broken defibrillator paddle—under the skin of its chest. With weak current, they induced ventricular fibrillation by stimulating the heart during the vulnerable period. Then, with a single, much stronger twenty-joule shock, they terminated the fibrillation and brought the dog back to life. To publicize their achievement, they made a movie showing a dog first collapsing unconscious in cardiac arrest, then getting shocked by an implantable defibrillator, and finally standing up and wagging its tail. When observers suggested the dog had been trained to fall down and stand up, Mirowski filmed additional sequences with simultaneous EKG tracings to prove that his dogs' hearts were indeed fibrillating. The film convinced many doctors that Mirowski was onto something with potentially great clinical benefits. In the spring of 1970, Earl Bakken of Medtronic visited Mirowski to inspect his apparatus. Mirowski performed a successful demonstration for his guest. Afterward, when Bakken asked what would have happened if the revived dog had not been defibrillated, Mirowski disconnected the defibrillator, put the dog back into ventricular fibrillation, and stood by as it quickly died.

In a monumental blunder, Bakken decided that Mirowski's device was not commercially viable. Since sudden death is essentially random, he wondered how Mirowski was going to identify patients most at risk. (Mirowski decided to focus on patients who had already survived cardiac arrest. Whether patients with heart disease but no history of cardiac arrest can benefit from an implantable defibrillator is a question that Mirowski was unable to answer and one that cardiologists are still grappling with.) Bakken also wondered how Mirowski was going to test his device. Would he have to put people into cardiac arrest to see if his apparatus worked? (The answer was yes.) Was that even ethical?

So Mirowski and his team continued on their own, undeterred and largely unfunded. On February 4, 1980, they finally did their first human test. The fifty-four-year-old California woman had had multiple episodes of cardiac arrest. In the operation, surgeons at the Johns Hopkins Hospital implanted an electrode in her superior vena cava and sutured a patch electrode to the surface of her left ventricle. They inserted the generator into her abdomen. (As was the case with some medical school cadavers, early pacemaker and defibrillator generators were installed in the abdominal cavity.) Then, to test the device, they put her into ventricular fibrillation. The device did not activate at first. For fifteen seconds, Mirowski and his colleagues watched spellbound as the woman went unconscious. They were getting ready to apply an external defibrillator to her chest when the implantable defibrillator finally fired. One shock was all it took to revive her. Though *The New England Journal of Medicine* had rejected Mirowski's first paper on his animal experiments, it quickly published his experience with his first three subjects in a paper called "Termination of Malignant Ventricular Arrhythmias with an Implanted Automatic Defibrillator in Human Beings." Five years later, in 1985, the Food and Drug Administration approved commercial production of the device.

•

Seventeen years after FDA approval, Jack, my patient, was ready to become a reluctant beneficiary of Mirowski's invention. Lightly sedated with midazolam and Ativan, he lay on a table in the cath lab, his head propped up on a foam wedge to help his breathing. He was relaxed and attentive. When I inserted a needle into his groin in preparation for the catheter, he seemed bemused, even tickled. "Oh my God, look, it's my blood!" he said.

I had a harder-than-usual time slipping the catheter into the right coronary artery. It turned out to be anomalous, originating from an unusual place. So Dr. Fuchs took over with a differently shaped catheter. "That's the way it is with me," Jack said, when I explained to him what was going on. "I'm an anomaly." Fortunately, the right coronary was clean. The left coronary, too, was mostly normal. There was small plaque in the midportion, but it was unlikely to cause any trouble, so we decided to leave it alone. When I told Jack that we were done with the angiogram, he told us to keep on working. "You can go on for another hour if you want." The scrub nurse laughed. Jack rather enjoyed being the center of attention. He seemed to appreciate an opportunity to be charming, even if it was on a surgical table.

We transferred Jack to a stretcher and rolled him over to the neighboring electrophysiology suite, where the beeper-sized defibrillator was going to be implanted. Under the intense ceiling lights, his hospital gown was removed. I started off by cleaning his chest with three different antiseptic soaps. Then I pressed a clear antibiotic-impregnated film onto his skin. Defibrillator infections are rare, less than one in a thousand, but when they occur, the device must be surgically removed, so we had to be extremely careful to keep the operating field germ-free. Before long, Jack was getting a milky-white anesthetic, enough so he wouldn't experience pain during the procedure but not so much that he could not breathe on his own.

Shapiro, the colorful electrophysiology attending, entered with flair. "Honey, I'm home," he boomed to the nurses. Together, we gowned, masked, and gloved. Then I tipped the table downward to put Jack's head below his legs so blood would fill his chest veins to make them more visible. Shapiro injected Novocain into the skin and soft tissue. "That hurt," Jack mumbled, and Shapiro told him to stop talking. "It's dangerous for you," he said, winking at me before increasing the rate of the anesthetic drip.

With an electrical knife, Shapiro made a two-inch incision on the left upper chest, close to the shoulder. He dissected through the layer of yellow fat with the blunt end of a pair of scissors, down to the glistening white fascial plane and then below the pectoral muscle, where he burrowed a pocket for the defibrillator. Because Jack was so thin, we wanted to put the device below the muscle so it wouldn't create too much of a bulge. I stood to one side, mostly watching. Occasionally, I was asked to cauterize a tiny bleeder, and so I'd pull out the electrical knife, releasing a thin wisp of blood smoke. Every few minutes, Shapiro would step back from the table and dance wildly to the song ("Roxanne," "Rock Lobster") on the radio.

Before long, Shapiro inserted a twenty-two-gauge needle into a chest vein, pulling back on the hub of the syringe until it suddenly gave way, filling the clear plastic column with maroon blood, a sign of low oxygen tension. He threaded a slippery guide wire, like a guitar string, through the bore of the needle and into the vein. When he knew it was safely in, he pulled out the needle. "Never let go of the wire," he said, and I nodded nervously. Shapiro threaded a plastic catheter over the wire and pulled the wire out of the vessel, leaving the catheter in place. Then he inserted a thin electrode through the hollow catheter and inched it forward into the heart. On the X-ray screen, it curved into the organ like a snake ready to strike. It buckled ever so slightly when it made contact with the inner surface of the right ventricle. Out came the catheter, leaving the electrode in place. Shapiro then placed a second wire through a large vein and onto the surface of the left ventricle. He slipped the generator, the size of a credit card but about a centimeter thick, into the pectoral pocket and connected it to the wires.

We were done. All that effort over the past several months, and Jack, my magnetic patient, had finally gotten his defibrillator. It was time to test the device by fibrillating Jack's heart. The Medtronic rep, a courtly, graying man who was there to help with the testing, called for me from across the room. "Step right up," he said, standing in front of a small computer. "Now you're going to kill your patient."

I was supposed to deliver stimuli to the heart during the vulnerable period to induce ventricular fibrillation. I pressed a few buttons on the keyboard to pace the heart three times and then deliver an extra impulse at a variable delay, trying to time the extra impulse into the vulnerable period to cause cardiac arrest. The stream of electrical pulses made cartoonish sounds, like Pac-Man gobbling dots. I started with an extra stimulus at 330 milliseconds. A few squiggles appeared on the screen, denoting a burst of disordered electrical activity, but the rhythm returned to normal. I repeated the test at 320, 310, and 300 milliseconds, with a similar result. But the next beat, at 290 milliseconds, did what we wanted. On the monitor, Jack's picket-fence heartbeat transformed into a sine wave oscillating at several different frequencies. It was ventricular fibrillation, the rhythm of death. "Here we go," the rep said excitedly. He started counting: "Five . . . ten . . . fifteen." The defibrillator was programmed to shock after eighteen cycles of the sine wave. Though Jack had been awake this whole time, when I looked over he was now unconscious. I heard a dull thump, as if someone had driven a fist into Jack's bony chest, and his body jumped ever so slightly off the table. The defibrillator had fired. On the screen, there was a spike and a pause, and then the EKG returned to normal. A nurse lightly slapped Jack's face. "Wake up," she said. "It's all over."

Afterward, I asked Shapiro what we would have done if the implantable defibrillator hadn't worked and external defibrillation was also ineffective. "It's happened before," he said. "You get these floppy hearts, and you induce fibrillation, and you can't always shock them out of it." He paused and started wiping down his hands. "It doesn't make us happy," he said, as if recalling a bad memory. He glanced at me once more. "It doesn't make us happy."

•

A couple of weeks later, I saw Jack in the clinic. He was wearing his bowler and a vintage blazer, looking even more stylish than usual. He said he was feeling better. There was more color in his face. He had gained some weight, too.

He had given up his magnets, which he could no longer apply to his body because they interfered with his defibrillator. (This was probably the reason he had resisted the device for so long, I realized.) I inspected the implantation site. It was red but dry and intact. There were small bandages covering the incision.

"The visiting nurse suggested more diuretic to treat the swelling in my legs," Jack said, hopping onto the exam table. "What do you think?" I couldn't help but smile. I had been recommending this for months. "I think that would be a good idea, Jack," I said.

He reminded me that before he left the hospital, he'd agreed to increase fosinopril, one of his heart medications. "But sometimes it makes me dizzy," he said. "Would it be all right if I cut the dose in half?" I started to laugh. Jack, once my most noncompliant patient, had become a convert to modern cardiology. To think that all it took was to bring him back from the dead.

But before I could say anything, Jack reminded me that doctors in the hospital had stopped his herbal supplements. "They did give me magnesium, but in the gluconate form, which you can't absorb," he said with irritation. As soon as he got home, he'd gone back to taking his usual nutraceutical cocktail. "I'm finally feeling better," he said. "I won't ever let that happen again."

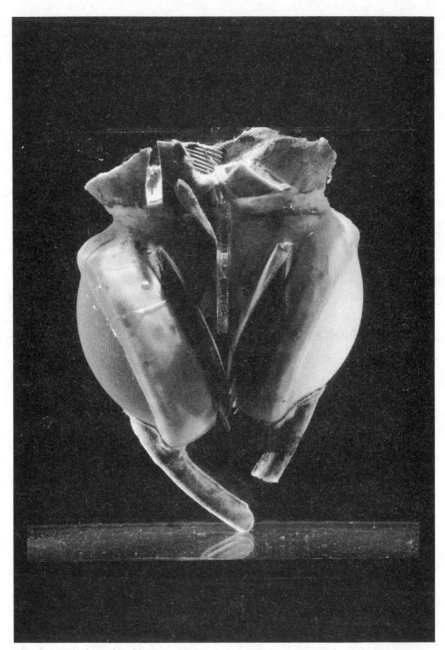

The first total artificial heart (Gift of Dr. Denton Cooley, Division of Medicine and Science, National Museum of American History, Smithsonian Institution. Reproduced by permission)

11

Replacement Parts

For a dying man [a heart transplant] is not a difficult decision . . . If a lion chases you to the bank of a river filled with crocodiles, you will leap into the water, convinced you have a chance to swim to the other side.
　　　　　　—Christiaan Barnard, South African surgeon

The mother had on red lipstick, thickly and haphazardly applied. Her eyes were swollen, her hair tied up in a bun. Tears had left tracks on her brown, pitted cheeks. When she saw me, the tears started up again.

Ravindra, her twenty-five-year-old son, was dying, and we both knew it. I'd been dreading the conversation we should already have had, and so apparently had she. Whenever I'd tell her that we needed to discuss her son's condition, she'd tell me to speak with her husband, Ravindra's father. He was a simple man, a salesman, who would sit quietly, square-jawed, even as his wife wailed in grief. When he could bear it no longer, he would put his arm around her and gruffly say, "Come on, woman, come on."

Curled up on a stretcher in the emergency room, their son was gulping air. His breathing had quickened over the past several days; that is why they had brought him in. Crusted mouth, sunken eyes, wasted temples: he rested unnaturally on the bedsheet, his body almost folding in on itself, a consequence of Friedreich's ataxia, a hereditary nerve disease that robs motor function of the arms and legs and, in its final stages, destroys the heart, too. On an echo, his heart wasn't so much beating as twisting, trying to expel its contents. Though he was an adult, he looked no older than a teenager. A tiny wisp of a mustache was all that distinguished him from the adolescent patients down the hall. At Christmas, I'd put up the money for an Xbox for him, as I'd done for my own son, Mohan. It was the only thing Ravindra wanted, but the family could not afford to buy one. Sadly, he never got to play with it. By the time the holidays rolled around, he was too debilitated, confined to a motorized wheelchair when he wasn't lying in bed. I remembered the embarrassed look on his face when his mother showed me pictures of him when he was younger. In one photograph, he was standing on a pier, a large body of water behind him, broad-shouldered in a red tank top. When I asked him if he liked the picture, he nodded without looking up. When a nurse asked if the pictures were really of him, he loudly grunted yes.

Now he was back in the hospital. He'd been admitted the previous month, too. When patients with heart failure begin to have frequent hospitalizations, it means their condition has taken a turn for the worse. It is a sign that the end is near.

I asked Ravindra to sit up so I could listen to his back. His father jumped out of his chair before I could correct myself. "He can't sit, Doc," he said apologetically.

"Yes, of course," I said, berating myself silently. I'd forgotten.

We pulled him up. His lung sounds were crackly. When I pressed on his distended belly, the veins in his neck popped out like straws. Typical symptoms of end-stage heart failure include shortness of breath, fatigue, nausea, and mental lassitude. Ravindra had all of them.

I put away my stethoscope and stepped back from the stretcher. His parents stared at me. "Don't let him die," his mother whispered, as if reading my thoughts. "We are not ready to say goodbye."

I asked Ravindra's father to step outside. In the hallway, we faced each other squarely. He had a trim beard. He worked part-time as a Hindu priest. Traces of red powder were still on his forehead.

"His heart is getting weaker," I said, not sure how to begin.

"It gets weaker and weaker until it finally stops?" he said. I nodded, not having the energy to disabuse him of this misconception. I could feel his desperation. I had a son, too.

I remembered the story he'd told me of how Ravindra got sick. "He used to pull his hair, bite his clothes," the father had recounted. "Schoolteacher said something not right with him." They took him to a pediatrician, who did a blood test. "I don't know where he sent it. Then we went to seven more places with seven more tubes of blood, and then they come up with this. They told us he will end up in a wheelchair. We didn't believe them, but they were 100 percent right. Everything what they say, we see today. Only thing they got wrong was they said he would live for fifteen years. He lived for twenty-five."

Now, facing me outside his dying son's room, he asked me the question I'd been dreading. "Can you give him a new heart?"

•

Many diseases have a common, final pathway. For heart disease, that final pathway is heart failure. In the most common form, the heart's contractions weaken because of damage—heart attacks, chemical, viral—resulting in a drop in blood flow and blood pressure. Because blood pressure determines oxygen delivery to vital organs, the body does all it can to keep the pressure up. Hormones are released that signal the heart to beat faster and the kidneys to retain water to increase blood volume (and therefore blood pressure). These hormones are a temporary fix, however. Cardiac output and blood pressure often do return to normal levels, but at a great cost. The body becomes congested as fluid accumulates and leaks into tissues. As patients become weaker and malnourished, protein levels also drop, keeping even less fluid inside the veins. Soon, water is everywhere, filling up soft tissues in the legs, abdomen, and lungs. The French writer Honoré de Balzac had congestive heart failure. According to Victor Hugo, his close friend, Balzac's legs resembled "salty lard." They were so waterlogged that doctors tried draining them by puncturing the tight, congested skin with metal tubes, resulting in gangrene, from which he died.

Though patients with heart failure are often literally drowning in their own fluids, their kidneys continue to limit water excretion, incorrectly perceiving a low blood volume because of inadequate blood flow. Treating congestive heart failure is a Sisyphean struggle. The more fluid that is removed with diuretic drugs, the more fluid-retaining hormones get activated. In the end, the therapy becomes its own enemy. Half of all patients with heart failure die within five years of receiving the diagnosis. For the most severe cases, like Ravindra's, the average survival is only a few months.

The definitive treatment for end-stage heart failure is a heart transplant. The field has progressed quickly over the past several decades. Today the survival rate after cardiac transplantation is about 85 percent at one year, nearly four times better than the average survival of patients treated with medications alone.

But as recently as the early 1960s, heart transplantation seemed like a pipe dream. Organ rejection and life-threatening infections posed prohibitive risks. By the second half of the decade, however, animal research had pointed a path toward human transplantation.

In the end, the race to transplant the first human heart was primarily between Dr. Christiaan Barnard at Groote Schuur Hospital in Cape Town, South Africa, and Dr. Norman Shumway at Stanford. The two surgeons had been residents under Walt Lillehei at the University of Minnesota. By many accounts, they'd had a frosty relationship. Shumway scorned Barnard's showmanship, his aggressiveness, his willingness to cut corners. Barnard, for his part, resented the way his Minnesota colleague viewed him as a foreigner born into poverty in a pariah country. However, they did share the inspiration of their great surgical mentors, who guided them throughout their careers. It was Owen Wangensteen, the surgical chief at Minnesota, who arranged for Barnard to get his first heart-lung machine at Cape Town in 1958. Before Barnard used it—in the first open-heart surgery in apartheid-era South Africa—he received a letter of encouragement from Lillehei. "Nice and simple," Lillehei advised his protégé, describing the kind of surgery Barnard should attempt first. "Nothing too fussy, nothing too flashy. I have every confidence in you."

Barnard was up against a great challenge. In the 1960s, the United States—Stanford in particular—was the mecca of transplant cardiology. Plus, Shumway had a great deal more experience with animal transplants, which he had helped pioneer. In 1959, he and Richard Lower, a Stanford resident, performed the first dog heart transplant. The recipient lived for eight days, demonstrating that an organ could be transplanted from one animal to another and continue to function. By 1967, about two-thirds of Dr. Shumway's research dogs were able to live for a year or more. In late 1967, he announced in an interview in *The Journal of the American Medical Association* that he was going to start a clinical trial at Stanford to perform the first heart transplant in a human. "Although animal work should and will continue," he said, "we are none the less at the threshold of clinical application." At that point, he had transplanted hearts into nearly three hundred dogs. Barnard had done about fifty.

But Shumway was at a disadvantage when it came to finding a human donor. American regulations at the time prohibited organ harvesting from brain-dead patients if their hearts were still beating. The heart had to stop completely before organs—including the heart—could be collected.* Barnard, on the other hand, was governed by more liberal South African laws—legislation that he himself had presciently advocated for—that allowed a neurosurgeon to confirm death if a patient showed no response to light or pain, a much lower bar than the one for his American counterpart.[†] By South African standards, once family consent was obtained, a transplant team could quickly harvest organs, including the heart, while they were still being perfused with blood.

It was a close race, but Barnard broke the transplant tape first, on December 3, 1967, thirty-four days before Shumway. His first patient, Louis Washkansky, a fifty-five-year-old grocer, received the heart of a young woman who had suffered brain damage after being hit by a car while crossing the road. He lived for eighteen days after the procedure, succumbing to a lung infection after his immune system was weakened by drugs to prevent organ rejection. Shumway had to content himself with doing the first adult heart transplant in the United States a month later, on January 6, 1968. His patient, a fifty-four-year-old steelworker, lived for two weeks before surrendering to what Shumway described as "a fantastic galaxy of complications," including gastrointestinal bleeding and sepsis.

Today, with the development of antirejection drugs, the long-term outcomes following heart transplantation are excellent. The median survival is probably greater than twelve years (fourteen, if the patient survives the first year). The success has

---

*This was the case in other countries as well. In 1968, a Japanese surgeon was charged with murder after removing a patient's heart while it was still beating to harvest it for transplant. The charges were eventually dropped, after six years of litigation, but heart transplants were outlawed in Japan—indeed, the very term "heart transplant" was taboo—until 1997, when brain death was officially recognized.

[†]Brain death as a legal definition of death wasn't widely accepted in the United States until 1981, when a presidential commission issued a landmark report on the subject.

been a mixed bag, however. Though many lives have been saved, many more have been lost while patients have waited for a viable organ. Only about 3,000 Americans receive a heart transplant each year, though roughly 4,000 are on the transplant list and perhaps ten times that number would benefit from a transplant if an organ were available. Despite public campaigns to increase organ-donor awareness, the number of available organs has remained relatively constant over the years (in part because of seat belt and motorcycle helmet laws that have resulted in fewer road fatalities). For this reason, heart transplants will never be the answer for the 250,000 or so patients in the United States with advanced heart failure. As the Vanderbilt University cardiologist Lynne Warner Stevenson put it, "Relying on transplants to cure heart failure is a bit like relying on the lottery to cure poverty."

Therefore, replacing the human heart with an off-the-shelf mechanical device has been the great ambition of cardiologists and cardiac surgeons for the past half century. At first glance, the obstacles seem insurmountable. Blood quickly coagulates when it encounters plastic or metal. Without adequate blood thinning, clots can be expelled from an artificial heart and course through the body, blocking arteries and causing strokes and other damage. An artificial heart also can never stop pumping, even temporarily, so without an internal battery to drive the device, power lines must travel into the body, posing the risk of infection. Moreover, even as recently as the late 1960s, a mechanical device had never been housed inside a human body in direct contact with the bloodstream. It was impossible to predict the consequences. And so, even a generation ago, building an artificial heart appeared preposterously wishful. But that didn't stop some from trying.

Willem Kolff, a Dutch physician, would be the first to succeed. The inventor of the artificial kidney, he moved on to a more vital organ when he performed the first artificial-heart replacement in an animal at the Cleveland Clinic in 1957. Kolff's organ held two balloon-like sacs filled with blood inside its plastic ventricles. Pressurized air filled the ventricles and compressed the balloons, thus forcing blood out in much the same way as from a beating heart. Kolff's subject, a dog, survived for approximately ninety minutes. A few years later, at a congressional hearing in 1963, Michael DeBakey, a distinguished surgeon at Baylor College of Medicine in Houston, called for federal investment to support research like Kolff's. "It is possible to completely replace the heart with an artificial [device], and animals have been known to survive as long as thirty-six hours," he told the legislators. This idea could reach "full fruition," he predicted, if there was funding to support more research, especially in bioengineering. DeBakey's appeal fell on receptive ears. American cardiovascular research had produced a steady stream of life-prolonging innovations over the previous decade, including the heart-lung machine, implantable pacemakers, and external and implantable defibrillators. Despite this progress, heart disease remained the number one killer in the country. Critics, such as Congressman John Fogarty, chairman of the House Appropriations Health Subcommittee—and a cardiac patient himself; he died of a heart attack in 1967—noted that millions were being spent to put a man on the moon. Why couldn't more money be invested to help Americans dying at home?

And so, in 1964, the National Institutes of Health started the Artificial Heart Program "with a sense of urgency," as an ad hoc committee advised, with the goal of putting a man-made heart into a human by the end of the decade.

On April 4, 1969, just before the decade ran out, the surgeon Denton Cooley, DeBakey's great rival at St. Luke's Episcopal Hospital in Houston, implanted the first artificial heart, made of polyester and plastic and powered by compressed air, into Haskell Karp, a forty-seven-year-old Illinois man suffering from end-stage heart failure. After the implant, which was supposed to provide only a few days of support, a frantic search

for a donor heart commenced. A compatible organ was identified three days later in Boston. The donor was put on a chartered
Learjet outfitted with a full medical team from Houston, but
on the flight home the plane's hydraulic system failed, and the
pilot was forced to make an emergency landing. Another jet
was dispatched, but by the time the donor arrived in Houston,
they had a problem; his heart was damaged. On the ambulance
ride to the hospital, the donor heart fibrillated, requiring electrical shocks and chest compressions to keep it pumping. It
was transplanted successfully, but Karp died thirty-two hours
after the operation.

Though $40 million of federal money had been spent over
almost a decade, many considered Cooley's attempt premature.
More research was needed to design surfaces that would not
create blood clots, as well as to develop an internal generator
so patients would not have to be hooked up to an external power
source. Through the 1970s, many refinements were made to
artificial-heart design, including changing the shape of the organ and developing more blood-compatible materials. In 1981,
Cooley tried again. This time, the artificial heart provided
thirty-nine hours of support, but again the patient died shortly
after heart transplantation.

Cooley's artificial hearts were intended as interim therapy,
a temporary bridge to heart transplantation. Neither was designed to be a long-term replacement. However, many patients
with end-stage heart failure do not qualify for transplantation
because of advanced age or coexisting medical conditions. Such
patients require permanent support or "destination therapy," a
bridge not to transplant but to eventual death.

The concept of permanent mechanical support was put
to the test a year after Cooley's second implant when a retired
dentist named Barney Clark was wheeled into an operating
room at the University of Utah Medical Center. Clark, who was
sixty-one, had end-stage heart failure caused by a viral infection. He had originally been scheduled for surgery on the

morning of December 2, 1982—coincidentally, almost exactly fifteen years after Christiaan Barnard's first heart transplant— but when his condition acutely worsened on the night of December 1, in the middle of a heavy snowstorm, his doctors decided to press ahead with the world's first permanent artificial heart. By the time the seven-hour operation was over, it had unleashed a blizzard of a different kind.

By all accounts, when Clark was hospitalized in late November, he was near the end of his life. For months he had suffered from intolerable shortness of breath, nausea, and fatigue. On Thanksgiving Day, family members had to carry him to the dinner table at his home in Seattle, but he was unable to eat. In the intensive care unit in Salt Lake City, he was placed in a dark room and visitation was restricted; doctors feared that any sort of excitement could precipitate ventricular fibrillation. William DeVries, the lead surgeon, was sure that "death appeared imminent within hours to days."

Because of his age and severe emphysema, Clark was not eligible for a heart transplant. When his doctors brought up the option of an artificial heart, Clark visited a laboratory at the University of Utah where calves had been kept alive for months with a Jarvik-7 device. The Jarvik-7 was developed in Utah by Robert Jarvik, an engineer working in the laboratory of Willem Kolff, who'd implanted the first artificial heart in a dog at the Cleveland Clinic in 1957 before moving his research enterprise to Salt Lake City. Though the Jarvik-7 carried Jarvik's name (because Kolff generously named his artificial hearts after the laboratory colleague who had worked on the most recent model), it relied on many of Kolff's original designs from the 1950s. The aluminum-and-plastic heart had two separate ventricles grafted with polyester sleeves to the native atria and great vessels and was powered by an air compressor that weighed almost four hundred pounds. The sight must have disturbed Clark because he told his doctors that he would take his chances with medical therapy. But worsening heart failure forced him to reconsider, and so in the early morning of December 2, Clark emerged from the operating room with plastic tubes coming out of his chest, connected to a refrigerator-sized machine. Though he was very much alive, his electrocardiogram was a flat line. His own heart had been removed from his body. The Jarvik-7 did its work.

DeVries and his colleagues could not have anticipated the intense worldwide interest in their experiment. Though I was only thirteen at the time, I still remember the daily news coverage. Teams of reporters and television crews swarmed the medical center, hankering for information about Clark's condition, even sneaking into the intensive care unit to check on him. The hospital cafeteria was transformed into a virtual press club, with hospital spokesmen providing twice-daily briefings. Clark's private struggle quickly became a public spectacle.

Though he opened his eyes and moved his limbs three hours after the operation, his subsequent course was rocky. On day 3, he underwent exploratory surgery because of air bubbles in his chest wall. On day 6, he suffered generalized seizures that left him in a coma. On day 13, his prosthetic mitral valve malfunctioned, and he had to go back to the operating room to have the left ventricle replaced. Many complications followed, including respiratory failure requiring a tracheostomy, kidney failure, pneumonia, and sepsis. On day 92, DeVries spoke with Clark in a videotaped interview. "It's been hard, hasn't it, Barney?" DeVries said. "Yes, it's been hard," Clark replied. "But the heart itself is pumping right along." It continued to pump until he finally succumbed to multi-organ failure on day 112.

Clark's Jarvik-7 became medicine's Sputnik; never before had a medical innovation sparked such furious debate, even a kind of national reckoning. Though some doctors viewed the experiment—two decades and $200 million in the making— as successful, most people were deeply disturbed by what they had witnessed. Some were repulsed that the human heart had been replaced by a machine made of metal and plastic. For them, the heart still carried special spiritual and emotional significance that made it impossible to replace with a man-made device. (Una Loy, Clark's wife, expressed this belief when she worried he might not still be able to love her.) Others felt Clark had not been adequately informed of the hazards of the artificial heart, even though the poor prognosis had been laid out and he had signed two consent forms—eleven pages, double-spaced—twenty-four hours apart to give him time to change his mind. (These concerns seem to ignore the fact that Clark viewed his participation as a sort of humanitarian mission. "It's been a pleasure to be able to help people," he said three weeks before he died. "And maybe you folks learned something.") Still others were troubled by the fact that Clark never left the hospital. He had survived for almost four months, they said. But had he really lived?

After Clark died, there was a period of public disenchantment with artificial organs. *The New York Times* dubbed artificial-heart research a kind of "Dracula" that was sucking money away from more worthwhile programs. After Clark, three more patients in the United States and one in Sweden were implanted with the Jarvik-7 as a permanent heart replacement. (The longest survivor was a man who lived for 620 days, much of it outside the hospital, but died of strokes and infections.) In 1985, three new artificial-heart models were introduced, including the Jarvik 7–70, which was smaller than its predecessor and powered by fluid, not pressurized air, so large tubes did not emanate from the body. The design, as Jarvik, the engineer, put it, "came from the understanding that people want a normal life and just being alive is not good enough." However, complications were severe, and most patients died within a few months. By the latter part of the decade, artificial hearts were back to being used almost exclusively as a bridge to heart transplantation. In 1990, the Food and Drug Administration issued a moratorium on the use of the Jarvik-7 device.

Though research began to focus on smaller, novel devices

that would assist the native heart, work continued on a total artificial heart. On July 2, 2001, the first fully contained artificial heart with no power lines was implanted in a fifty-eight-year-old man at Jewish Hospital in Louisville, Kentucky. The hydraulically powered device, made of titanium and polyurethane, the stuff of skateboard wheels, was about the size of a grapefruit and had a battery that could be recharged through intact skin, obviating the need for an external power source. The patient lived for five months before dying of a stroke.

Research on artificial hearts continues today. Nearly a hundred patients have been supported with the most recent model, CardioWest. The long-term support record is held by an Italian patient, who survived for 1,373 days before a successful heart transplant. But significant obstacles remain, including infection, bleeding, clotting, and strokes. The most recent devices produce continuous blood flow, so patients emerge from the operating room without a pulse. Continuous-flow devices are simpler than devices that send out pulses of blood, mimicking the native heart. They don't require valves and have fewer moving parts, resulting in less wear and tear. They still pump blood, of course, but the flow is constant, not periodic. Incredibly, humans, we now know, can live for long periods without pulsatile blood flow. However, continuous-flow hearts produce their own complications. They chew up blood cells because of the shear forces generated by the device and may strip the blood of clotting proteins. For unclear reasons, they cause tiny blood vessels that are prone to rupture to sprout up in the gastrointestinal tract, so patients often bleed internally. They can also cause degeneration in arterial walls and scarring. Continuous blood flow is antithetical to the way that humans, pulsatile beings, evolved. Though continuous flow can keep us alive, it alters our physiology in idiosyncratic and unpredictable ways.

Not long ago, I took a tour of a cardiothoracic surgical unit at Advocate Christ Medical Center, a major tertiary care facility just outside Chicago. My guide, an Indian cardiologist in

her sixties, had started one of the top artificial-heart programs
in the country in Louisville, Kentucky, before moving to
Advocate Christ. She took me on a tour of a twenty-five-bed
unit where patients were getting all manner of cardiac support,
from balloon pumps to ventricular assist devices to transplanted
hearts. I asked her what she thought about the prospects for
a total artificial heart. "It's an evolving field," she said carefully,
"but the complications are really troubling." She told me about
one of her patients with intractable arrhythmias who received
an artificial heart. His pain and suffering with it were so great
that his family sued the hospital and his doctors after he died.

We passed by a patient on a ventilator and dialysis machine;
she'd had a large myocardial infarction and was now being
supported by ventricular assist devices on both sides of her heart.
The multiple consoles surrounded her like a pack of animals.
"After so many years of study, I've concluded that the best thing
we can do for most of our patients is to give them medicine,"
the cardiologist told me. "Of course, we need mechanical devices for patients who are crashing and burning, but for most
of our patients the technology still has too many problems."

The workhorse of mechanical support for heart-failure patients today is not the artificial heart but the left-ventricular assist device (LVAD), which attaches to the native heart, pumping
blood directly out of the left ventricle and into the aorta, thus
essentially bypassing the failing organ. Approved by the FDA
for both permanent and bridge therapy, LVADs have become a
lifesaving option for end-stage heart-failure patients. Between
2006 and 2013, more than ten thousand patients, including
Vice President Dick Cheney, received LVADs for cardiac support. Unfortunately, LVADs are still not an option for patients
with severe failure of both right and left ventricles. For such
patients, like Barney Clark, a permanent artificial heart may
still be the best hope. For now, it remains a dream, but not
quite the pipe dream it was in 1982, when a soft-spoken dentist from Seattle decided to go first.

•

It wasn't easy telling Ravindra's father that there was nothing more I could offer, that his son was not eligible for a mechanical or a human heart because neither would change his poor prognosis. But I believe he already knew. "The things that are important to my wife are not so important to me," he said.

"What is important to you?" I asked.

"All the pain he going through." His lips quivered before his face tightened up again. "I don't want him to suffer no more. He have suffered enough."

Unfortunately, there was more suffering to come. Over the next several days, Ravindra had terrible leg pains. I wasn't sure why—poor blood flow to the muscles, perhaps—but I couldn't leave him in such agony. I put him on a morphine drip to keep him sleepy and as comfortable as possible. I made sure his father signed a do-not-resuscitate form. It didn't mean we wouldn't do everything in our power to help Ravindra, just that at the end we would let him go peacefully. His father understood. He was ready for the ordeal to end, both for himself and for his son.

On morphine, Ravi went in and out of consciousness. He'd doze off and then open his eyes in a panic, before closing them and sinking back into a fog. At times he displayed "agonal" breathing—loud gulps of air followed by periods of apnea, or no breathing—a pattern that frequently heralds death. His lungs made deep, guttural groans, like a foghorn, so congested were they with fluid. Sometimes he'd writhe with pain, mouth foaming, teeth clenched, a tight scowl on his face. Other times he would scream out, "Mom, help me, Mom!" His mother massaged his legs, day and night, and mumbled prayers and wept. As a doctor and just as a father, I found it a terrible thing to witness.

He died one morning before I made rounds. When I got upstairs, the door to his room was closed, but I could still hear the commotion inside. A nurse offered to go in with me, but I told her it wasn't necessary. As a heart-failure specialist, I'd experienced enough death to fill up a lifetime. Once, it was difficult to witness the grief of loved ones. But my heart had been hardened, and this was no longer that time.

At the bedside was a wooden table with drawers, and on the far side of the room were dark gray curtains framing windows overlooking the parking lot. Ravi's mother was smothering his face with kisses, talking almost robotically, as her grief erupted in ever more intense swirls. "No more, no more, my son is gone! Oh, my Father, my loving son no more!"

A relative sitting on the flower-patterned couch tried to comfort her. "He suffer too much, sister," she said. "It's God's choice. He will come back again in a nice body."

The father came over and hugged me. He was wearing an overcoat, though it was spring. "She will cool down," he whispered, referring to his wife. "She seen how he suffered."

"Oh, my son be punished and punished," the mother wailed. "He said, 'Mom, I'm dying, I'm dying, I can't breathe!' I told God to leave him, I would take him at 50 percent. But He wouldn't even give me that."

There wasn't much I could offer at that moment, so I said I would come back and exited. The father followed me out. In the hallway, he asked me what was next.

The body would be taken to the morgue, I explained. The funeral home would call to arrange for transportation. He seemed calm talking about the arrangements. Then his cell phone rang. He put in the earpiece. "Hello . . . yes, my son no more." And finally, he broke down, too.

PART III

Mystery

12

Vulnerable Heart

When the heart is affected it reacts on the brain; and the state of the brain again reacts . . . on the heart; so that under any excitement there will be much mutual action and reaction between these, the two most important organs of the body.
—Charles Darwin, *The Expression of the Emotions in Man and Animals* (1872)

The morgue was inside Brooks Brothers. I was standing at the corner of Church and Dey, right next to the rubble of the World Trade Center, when a policeman shouted that doctors were needed at the menswear emporium inside the building at One Liberty Plaza. Bodies were piling up there, he said, and another makeshift morgue on the other side of the rubble had just closed. I volunteered and set off down the debris-strewn street.

It was the day after the attack. The smoke and stench of burning plastic were even stronger than on Tuesday. The street was muddy, and because I was stupidly wearing clogs, the mud soaked my socks.

I arrived at the building. In the lobby, exhausted firefighters and their German shepherds were sitting on the floor amid broken glass. A soldier stood at the entrance to the store, where a crowd of policemen hovered. "No one is allowed in the morgue except doctors," he shouted.

I entered reluctantly through a dark curtain. Cadavers had always made me feel queasy, ever since those dog days in the anatomy lab in St. Louis. In the near corner was a small group of doctors and nurses, and next to them was an empty plastic stretcher. Behind the group was a wooden table where a nurse and two medical students were sitting grim-faced, looking like some sort of macabre tribunal. Brooks Brothers shirts were neatly folded in cubbyholes in the wall. They were covered in grime, but you could still make out the reds and oranges and yellows. In the far corner, next to what looked like a blown-out door, was a pile of orange body bags, about twenty of them. Soldiers were standing guard. In the store's dressing room were stacks of unused body bags.

The group was discussing the protocol for how to handle the bodies. A young female doctor said that she didn't think anyone should sign any forms, lest someone think that we had certified the contents of the bags, which we were not qualified to do. That, she said, was up to the medical examiner. Someone asked whether a separate body bag was needed for each body part, but no one knew the answer. The leader of the group was a man in his fifties. I looked at his badge. It read "PGY-3." He was a third-year resident, which meant that I was probably the most experienced doctor in the room, a thought that deeply disturbed me. I had been a cardiology fellow for only a couple of months.

At this point, some National Guardsmen brought in a body bag and laid it on the stretcher. The female doctor unzipped it and inspected the contents. "Holy Mother of God," she said, and she turned away. In the bag was a left leg and part of a pelvis, to which a penis was still attached. The leg itself hardly seemed injured, but the pelvic stump was beefy red and broken intestines were hanging out of it. A pants pocket was partially covering the pelvis and was emptied of change; this pocket was put in a separate bag. A policeman said that part of the victim's body had been brought in earlier, along with a cell phone.

That was actually good news. If the victim had the numbers of family members on his speed dial, he would be quickly identified. But identification wasn't my job. Processing was.

After five minutes, the bag was zipped up. The older male doctor, who had been working there for hours, said he had to leave. The other doctor also said she had to get away for about an hour. "Are you a physician?" she asked me. "Yes," I replied. "Great," she said. "You can take over." Then she started giving me instructions on how to catalog the body parts. Basically, I had to call out the contents of each bag to a nurse, who would write them down on a form. That was it.

I was in a fog. Suddenly I was in charge, but I wasn't a pathologist. I was just improvising. I recalled my friends who had done medical clerkships in Africa. They had told me of the terrible tragedies and deep frustration of not having proper medical supplies. But we were not suffering from a lack of supplies. This was not third-world medicine. It was netherworld medicine, without rules.

Another body bag came in. This one had a spleen, some intestines, part of a liver. After sifting through the bag's contents, I began to feel ill. I walked past headless mannequins and out into the smoke-filled air.

Our triage center had been set up in a firehouse within yards of the World Trade Center plaza. From here, the destruction was even more profound. Bombed-out cars, coated with an inch of cement dust, lined the muddy streets. Steel beams of the demolished towers stood up in the rubble like butts in an ashtray. Giant hoses and wires coiled from the buildings. Everywhere there were shattered windows and broken glass. The ground was strewn with paper and abandoned shoes, as if people had literally vanished in their tracks. Dr. Abramson, the Israeli echo chief who had accompanied me downtown, gazed at the carnage. "I thought I had seen every-thing," he said softly.

Our center was equipped with supplies—oxygen tanks, crates of foodstuffs—that had been ferried down by ambulance. A fire ladder served as a scaffold for bags of fluid. Twenty or so doctors and nurses staffed the different "departments": trauma, burns and injuries, wounds and fractures. I was in asthma and chest pain. We treated firefighters suffering from smoke inha-lation, giving them oxygen to breathe and albuterol mist to help open their airways. But otherwise things were eerily quiet.

On my way downtown the previous afternoon with a cara-van of doctors from Bellevue, I had braced myself to confront throngs of seriously injured people. But there was no one around except rescue workers. "Where are all the patients?" I blurted out when I arrived, thinking they might be at a different location.

"They're all dead," a colleague replied.

Now we sat in the haze, ash still falling like snow, trading stories. A physician told me he happened to be standing out-side the first tower when it collapsed. "I ran under a bridge," he said. "There was huge debris falling all around me. Every step I took, I kept saying to myself, 'I can't believe I'm not dead yet; I can't believe I'm not dead yet.'" Then he began hearing strange thuds. Those, a firefighter told him, were people jump-ing off buildings.

We sat for hours, waiting for something to happen. Then, in the early afternoon, word came that a victim, a young woman, had been found alive in the rubble. An American flag was hoisted at the site, and rescue workers began the painstak-ing work of extricating her. By late afternoon, about fifty doc-tors and other volunteers had formed a human chain from the street to the top of the rubble, several stories high, and were passing down the debris, piece by piece. Two large cranes with huge jaws then took the shrapnel and transferred it to waiting trucks.

I stayed until evening, hoping to help in some way, but I'd spent the better part of two days at the site, away from my worried wife, and I was exhausted. They were still working when I left.

For weeks after I returned to work that fall, the smell of dead bodies wafted from the morgue tents set up at First and Twenty-Ninth, outside Bellevue. I had been cutting through the street to get to conferences at the main hospital, but no more. Then, one day, I heard that the victim who'd been saved at Ground Zero was on the cardiac arrhythmia service, and not because of her broken leg. After her rescue, recurrent ventricular arrhythmias inexplicably set in, causing her to keep passing out. Medications couldn't suppress the arrhythmias, psychological counseling hadn't helped, and surgical options, including an implantable defibrillator, were being considered. By the late fall, she was on the catheterization table as electrophysiologists at Bellevue tried to figure out what had gone wrong inside her heart.

•

Heart rhythms are strongly influenced by emotional states. But how do emotions trigger rhythm disturbances? How does psychological injury disrupt the heart of a traumatized young woman that has beaten a billion times without fail? Bernard Lown, co-recipient of the Nobel Peace Prize for his work with International Physicians for the Prevention of Nuclear War, performed some of the seminal studies exploring such questions. As a high school student, Lown was fascinated by psychiatry, but in medical school he quickly became disenchanted by the subjective nature of the discipline. However, his fundamental interest in mind-body interactions persisted throughout his career. As a cardiologist in the 1960s, he decided to investigate whether psychological stress could trigger sudden cardiac death. In his earliest experiments, he studied ventricular fibrillation in anesthetized mice. To predispose the animals to fibrillation, Lown experimentally blocked a coronary artery, causing a small heart attack. He found that 6 percent of his animals developed ventricular fibrillation because of the coronary occlusion. However, Lown discovered that fibrillation occurred ten times more frequently when regions in the brain that mediate anxiety were electrically stimulated at the same time the coronary artery was occluded. Lown and his colleagues later found that they did not have to stimulate the brain to produce a fatal arrhythmia. Stimulating autonomic nerves that mediate blood pressure and heartbeat largely did the same thing.

But what Lown really wanted to show was that psychological stress by itself could trigger dangerous arrhythmias. He decided to study premature ventricular contractions (PVCs) in dogs. These extra heartbeats are often a precursor of fatal arrhythmias because they can strike during the vulnerable period of the cardiac cycle. PVCs indicate that the heart is in an excited and, therefore, vulnerable state. For the psychological stress, Lown put each dog in two different environments: a cage, in which the animals were essentially left undisturbed; and a sling, in which they were suspended, paws just off the ground, and received a single small electrical shock on three consecutive days. When the dogs were later returned to these two environments, Lown observed a remarkable difference. Animals placed in the cage appeared normal and relaxed. However, when they were transferred to the sling, they became restless, and their heartbeat and blood pressure went up. The rate of PVCs rose dramatically, too. Even months later, the memory of the minor sling trauma was deeply embedded in the dogs' brains and profoundly affected cardiac reactivity. These findings, Lown writes in his book *The Lost Art of Healing*, demonstrated that psychological stress, already known to be a risk factor for coronary artery disease, can substantially increase susceptibility to malignant arrhythmias, too.

Later, working with psychiatrists at the Brigham and Women's Hospital in Boston, Lown's team found that survivors of sudden arrhythmias often experience acute psychological stress preceding their cardiac arrest. Nearly 1 in 5 of a group of 117 patients suffered public humiliation, marital separation, bereavement, or business failure in the twenty-four hours prior to their attacks. Moreover, Lown and his colleagues showed that medications that block sympathetic nervous system activity, such as beta-blockers, protected patients from those arrhythmias. Meditation largely did the same thing.

Lown's research confirmed for the first time that emotional stress can initiate life-threatening arrhythmias. This conclusion is now widely accepted in medicine. We all agreed, for example, that post-traumatic stress was exacerbating the arrhythmias in the young woman rescued at Ground Zero. But in the months after 9/11, I learned a remarkable corollary to Lown's observations: not only are arrhythmias triggered by psychological trauma but they (or at least their treatment) can *cause* it as well. Such stress can then feed back onto the heart, creating a malignantly vicious cycle. The mind-heart link, in other words, goes both ways. One night in November, two months after the attacks, I got to see this up close.

•

I met Lorraine Flood on a rainy evening in the faculty dining room at NYU Medical Center, where about twenty patients with implantable cardiac defibrillators had assembled for a support-group meeting. In June 1998, eight years after her first heart attack on the eve of her son's wedding, Flood underwent an hour-long operation to implant a pager-sized defibrillator under the skin of her left chest. Like most patients, she was told that the device would monitor her heartbeat and apply a shock if the rhythm degenerated into something dangerous. "I was so relieved," Flood told me that night. "I used to worry, 'If something happens, I may not survive it.'" But then her defibrillator started working.

Flood was sitting with her husband, Al, with whom she had driven out from Colonia, New Jersey, where he was a bank executive and she owned a travel agency. She was a tall seventy-one-year-old woman with a regal bearing and salon-done blondish hair. I asked her why she had come to the meeting. "I've had a horrible time," she replied. "I still wake up every morning and pray to God and say, 'Lord, please, no shocks today. Please, no shocks today.'"

They started a few weeks after her implant, when she began to have arrhythmias that caused her defibrillator to fire. "I used to see this bluish-white light, and that was my warning I was going to get shocked," she said. She would quickly sit down and then feel the device discharge into her chest. "Nobody told me what it would be like. Oh, they said you'd feel a little something, but they never told me it was like a donkey rearing his hind legs and just with all the power he has hitting you right in the chest with full force—bang!"

Once, she was shocked sixteen times in nine days. "I was sitting on the couch when I started to get the shocks. I screamed like a banshee. My poor housekeeper didn't know what to do. She ran upstairs and got me a bathrobe and slippers to go to the hospital. I said, 'Catherine, I can wear clothes!'"

On the phone with her doctor, she was jolted by another intense shock. "I have always had a high threshold for pain—I never take Novocain at the dentist's—but I just couldn't handle it."

One afternoon, she was at her grandson's preschool when she saw the bluish-white light. "I felt it was warning me that I better get out of the room so I don't frighten the children," she recalled. She went into a bathroom, where she got what she described as a "mild shock." Later, when her doctors checked, they said the defibrillator hadn't fired. "They said it was a phantom shock," Flood said.* "But no one can tell me it wasn't re-

---

*Some patients experience what they describe as a shock; however, device interrogation shows no record of a shock being delivered. This condition has been termed phantom shock.

lated to the defibrillator. I've been shocked enough times to know what it was." Flood's defibrillator was adjusted to make it less sensitive to arrhythmias, but she continued to feel nervous, increasing the likelihood of future shocks.

She stopped going to work and hired a full-time driver. She stopped going out with friends or singing in the church choir and eventually resigned from the school board. She had tickets to *The Lion King* on Broadway but didn't use them because she was afraid of getting shocked during the performance. "Dr. Shapiro said to me, 'So what if you scream in the middle of the play? You'll scream, and then you'll watch the rest of the play.' But I couldn't do it."

Flood soon developed a Pavlovian fear of places where she had been shocked. One was her shower stall. "It once threw me against the wall of the shower," she said. "Well, you never saw anyone leave that shower so fast. I had shampoo in my hair, suds all over my body, and I ran into my bedroom screaming, and Al came running in. It was terrible." She started using her husband's bathtub. "I couldn't even look at the shower; that's how frightened I was," she said. "Then I decided, 'Lorraine, this is ridiculous.' One day I opened the shower door and put the water on. But I couldn't go in. I just watched the water."

Her constant fretfulness put a strain on her family. "I think my husband considered me a little cuckoo," Flood said. I asked her husband, a tall man with white hair and a patrician face, about this. He chose his words carefully. "It is a little hard for me to understand how paranoid she is with it," he admitted.

At a neighboring table, Mohammed Siddiqui, a well-dressed man in his late fifties, was sitting quietly with his wife, Anjali, waiting for the meeting to get started. Siddiqui said he had joined the support group three years prior, after his defibrillator was implanted, but it wasn't until the previous March that he had gotten shocked for the first time, in the passenger seat of his Nissan while his wife was driving. "It lifted up his whole body," his wife said. "He jumped in front of me. He was looking at me so strange I thought I must be going the wrong way."

That shock was followed by two others over the next ten days, including one while he was sleeping. When doctors checked, they said his defibrillator was responding appropriately to irregularities in his heartbeat and that he shouldn't worry. But instead of feeling reassured, he found himself constantly worrying about the next shock. Once an executive at a land-development company, he stopped driving because he was afraid of getting shocked on the road and having an accident. He avoided leaving his home and indefinitely postponed a visit to his family abroad. He lost ten pounds and started to feel chronically weak. He had what appeared to be classic post-traumatic stress disorder, with nightmares and recurrent thoughts about the event. His palpitations, his wife said, had only increased since the 9/11 attacks.

I walked over to the buffet table, where Dr. Shapiro, who had invited me to the meeting, was chewing on a chicken skewer. He had just gotten out of a procedure and was still wearing blue scrubs. "I see you've met Mr. Siddiqui," he said with a smirk. I told him what Siddiqui had said. Shapiro shrugged, seemingly at a loss for words. "I can't explain it," he said. "How can a shock make you weak for nine months?"

The meeting, Shapiro explained, was intended for people to open up about their defibrillators. Since the 9/11 attacks, he said, patients were reporting more defibrillator shocks than ever, probably because of increased psychological stress. The rate of ventricular arrhythmias in patients with implantable defibrillators had more than doubled. One patient of his, he said, was so disturbed after getting repeatedly shocked that she held a séance at her home to rid it of "evil spirits." Another had actually made Shapiro turn off his defibrillator. "He said he'd rather allow his life to end than deal with the pain and frequency of those shocks." Shapiro mentioned the young woman who was rescued at Ground Zero. No treatment for her arrhythmias had worked. The next step was probably a complex radio-frequency ablative procedure in her right ventricle.

Shapiro told me that his own father had gotten a defibrillator after a series of heart attacks. After the implant, his father's heart inexplicably went into incessant arrhythmias, an "electrical storm," and he was shocked eighty-five times in three hours. Traumatized, he couldn't sleep for weeks. "But I kept telling him the defibrillator was a good thing, that it was doing what it was supposed to," Shapiro said. "It was allowing him to see his grandchildren."

•

In the annals of dying, sudden arrhythmic death is something of a paradox: it is at once the most desirable way to die and the most feared. Sudden fatal arrhythmias are the leading cause of cardiovascular mortality across the world. Millions die of them every year, and most victims, like both my grandfathers, never even make it to the hospital. Most sudden cardiac deaths will leave loved ones bereft. But some will leave only gratitude for a merciful end.

Even as recently as thirty years ago, sudden arrhythmic death used to be greeted with almost total helplessness. Remember old movies in which a businessman slumps at his desk and a co-worker puts two fingers on his carotids and then pronounces him dead? The camera treated these deaths with an almost comical dispassion, as if they were fated, and this reflected society's powerlessness in the face of this killer. But things have changed since Michel Mirowski invented the implantable defibrillator. In 2016, about 160,000 defibrillators were implanted in the United States, more than double from a decade ago. The population of eligible patients has expanded, too—from actual survivors of cardiac arrest to patients like Jack, my magnetic patient, who are only at an increased risk of it.

Today Mirowski's invention is tiny (nine defibrillators would fit on this page), nearly foolproof, and highly effective.

The batteries last almost a decade and can be surgically replaced. Though it costs approximately $40,000 to implant one, considering that defibrillators often extend patients' lives by three years or more, the procedure in many cases is a bargain.

But all medical technology carries a different price. Artificial hearts cause blood clots and disabling strokes. Dialysis saves lives but often results in painful, even life-threatening, infections. For implantable defibrillators, designed to deliver peace of mind, one of the biggest downsides, paradoxically, is fear.

A few weeks before the support-group meeting, a senior cardiology fellow and I were called to the bedside of a twenty-four-year-old man, a professional basketball player in Europe, who had just been shocked for the first time by a defibrillator implanted earlier that day. He had been admitted to Bellevue a few days prior after passing out in practice; his doctors had identified a genetic heart abnormality. He was a muscular, intimidating man who was whimpering in pain when we arrived. His girlfriend wanted to know why the defibrillator had fired. My colleague and I "interrogated" the device with a special computer and found that it had delivered an "inappropriate" shock—meaning that it thought his heart was fibrillating when it was not. We made some adjustments. "Try not to worry," I said to the patient, who looked shell-shocked, as we were getting ready to leave. "If you get shocked in the future, you will have needed it." His girlfriend wanted to know if he could still play basketball. Would the defibrillator fire if a pass hit him in the chest or if his heart rate sped up during a game? It was unlikely, the senior fellow replied, but he conceded that it wasn't impossible. The patient thanked us, and we left. Somehow I knew he was never going to step on the court again.

•

A few months after her implant, Lorraine Flood went to her first support-group meeting. "I thought perhaps the stories I would hear from other people would help me," she said. She was surprised at how well the other patients were coping: going to their jobs, going on vacations, getting on with their lives. It was inspirational but a bit dispiriting, too, because she thought some people at the meeting were in denial. "Sometimes I had the impression that people weren't opening up," Flood told me, "that they weren't 100 percent honest about how painful a shock can be. One lady I befriended got shocked for the first time in a bank. She said, 'It was nothing.' Well, it's not nothing."

While the support group made Flood determined to get on with her life, her anxiety continued. Pretty soon, she was having full-blown panic attacks, which only worsened her arrhythmias. One evening when she was home alone, she suddenly experienced an overwhelming fear that her defibrillator was about to go off. She started sweating. She went to her neighbor's house; in his driveway there was a motion sensor wired to a lamp. When it went off, so did Flood. "I was screaming, crying uncontrollably, pounding on the door, tearing at my hair," she said. "I'm the type who needs everything to be in place, and I looked like something the cat dragged in."

Like many patients with post-traumatic stress disorder, she started taking Ativan, which helped. But one night, lying in bed, she saw a man in a black suit and a hat standing at the foot of her bed. Hallucinations are an uncommon side effect, but that was it for the Ativan.

Psychologists have come up with two theories to explain the post-traumatic stress disorder after implantable defibrillator shocks. The first, classical conditioning, refers to the psychological pairing of a previously neutral stimulus (such as taking a shower) with a noxious one (painful shock) so that they elicit the same fearful response. As in Flood's case, as well as for other patients at the support-group meeting—and, presumably, the young woman who survived at Ground Zero—fear can heighten arousal and result in even more arrhythmias and shocks. The fear subserves itself.

The second theory derives from experiments in which dogs were repeatedly subjected to electrical shocks. Compared with controls, animals that are powerless to regulate their shocks become physically exhausted and quickly cease to struggle, despite being given opportunities to avoid the shocks. Researchers have concluded that animals acquire a state of "learned helplessness," like the wild rats trapped in water-filled jars in Curt Richter's experiments described in chapter 1. Humans who experience frequent shocks develop a similar response.

The key to avoiding such a hopeless state is to take away the element of surprise. Rats repeatedly shocked without warning develop stomach ulcers, a sign of intense arousal. However, rats that can predict when they will be shocked because of a warning buzzer develop significantly fewer ulcers. Moreover, rats that can prevent some shocks by pressing a lever develop fewer ulcers than those that receive the same number of shocks but have no control over them. Ulcers are further reduced when the rats, after pressing the lever, are given a signal that the shock has been successfully prevented. In other words, predictability, control, and feedback about the effectiveness of coping all reduce shock-induced stress.

Piggybacking on such research, researchers at Wake Forest University investigated how to mitigate the startle response of humans to sudden defibrillator shocks. They delivered 150-volt shocks to the arms of twenty volunteers and asked them to rate the pain. Some shocks were delivered alone; others following a tiny, painless "pre-pulse" so subjects were prepared. The pre-pulsed shocks were rated less painful than the ones applied without warning. The analgesic effect was greatest in the subjects who felt the most pain to begin with.

However, nothing has proved more effective for anxious patients than simply reducing the number of shocks they receive. Reprogramming a defibrillator to make it less sensitive to arrhythmias is the mainstay of treatment. Most patients are also put on an anti-arrhythmic drug, like amiodarone, which can have serious side effects like lung and thyroid problems but which most cardiologists find acceptable if it prevents the occasional errant shock and subsequent psychological cascade. Patients also often work with a clinical psychologist who specializes in shock-induced anxiety and provides cognitive-behavioral therapy. Many (like Flood) require antianxiety medications or antidepressants. For some, the best treatment is simply refraining from the activities that induce the shocks in the first place— for example, the patient who kept getting shocked during vigorous sex. (His partner claimed to feel it, too.)

But despite efforts to make them more user-friendly, defibrillators, like any medical technology, are always going to involve a compromise: What are you willing to give up to live a little longer? Ultimately, I think my maternal grandfather died the right way for him; he wasn't a burden on his family, and he was walking and talking until the very end, listening to the BBC every morning. He wouldn't have wanted to live with a donkey in his chest ready to kick him at any moment. A defibrillator might have given him another year or two. But what would he have traded for the extra time?

•

Not long after our meeting, I went out to New Jersey to see how Lorraine Flood was doing. It was a cold, drizzly December evening. Her two-story home in Colonia was on an upscale, tree-lined cul-de-sac. We sat down in her living room, where she had laid out a generous spread of shrimp cocktail and fruit salad. Dressed in tan slacks and a cream-colored sweater, she looked calm, at peace. I could hear the sounds of soft jazz coming from upstairs. "I got shocked over there," she said, pointing to a rocking chair. "I still can't sit on it."

Though her fear was not as incapacitating as it once was, she said, it was still a daily ritual. She still went "panicville" when a cell phone came near her. (The fear that a cell phone could make a defibrillator go haywire is common among patients, but unfounded.) "There are days the defibrillator is constantly on my mind," she confided. "Sometimes I feel my heart thumping, turning, going topsy-turvy. It frightens me because I'm not sure if it means I'm about to get shocked. At times like these, I forget I'm supposed to be a big girl and overcome it."

When the fear hit, she used simple techniques to divert her thoughts. She sang songs to herself that she learned when she was a girl. She chanted a Sanskrit mantra that she learned in her younger days as a yoga instructor. And she prayed.

Flood had started driving again, but she said she wouldn't go more than four miles from her house, the radius encompassing her office, the shopping mall, and her church. (When she had to go longer distances, a driver took her.) She was, however, back to taking showers every day. "But even now, when I go in the shower, I say to myself, I better face this way in case I get a shock, so I won't fall out the shower door."

As hard as she tried to overcome it, the fear of being shocked still occasionally unnerved her. "If you knew me before, I was such a happy-go-lucky free spirit," she said. "I'm very reserved now, very cautious. I'm afraid to do things."

In the end, I wondered, was the defibrillator worth it? "Yes," she said, "because I feel it could give me another six months or a year." Then she paused and added, "Every once in a while, my mind runs rampant, thinking that this is going to be my last day. I say to the Lord, 'If it's my time, let me go in my sleep, please.' "

•

A couple of years ago, I finally took my children to see the 9/11 Memorial in downtown Manhattan. For more than a decade, I'd avoided reading almost anything about the 9/11 attacks, so I had no idea what to expect. Approaching the main square, near where I had cataloged body parts at Brooks Brothers, I started to feel queasy. My armpits became moist, and my heart started to race. A crowd was packed at the viewing wall, surrounding the granite reflecting pool where the South Tower had once stood. I thought once again of the young woman with arrhythmias who was rescued the day after the attack. I never did find out what happened to her. Maybe her arrhythmias eventually responded to medications (or meditation). Maybe she underwent the radio-frequency procedure that Shapiro had mentioned, or even surgery to cut the sympathetic nerves that mediate the heart's response to emotional stress. More likely, she was implanted with a defibrillator to protect her from her heart's meandering vortices. Whatever the case, I wondered whether she was still alive to see the monument. We pushed our way through a gap in the mass of people. I pulled my children up to the stone wall. And then I saw it: the black stone, the bottomless pit, into which water swirled. It looked like a reentrant spiral wave, the signature of a heart's death. I closed my eyes. My head was spinning.

13

A Mother's Heart

In certain circumstances death may come like a thief in
the night to a susceptible person living with circulatory
conditions that approach the danger line.
—John A. MacWilliam, *British Medical Journal* (1923)

My mother loved to sleep. Sleep was her balm for the daily ir-
ritations of an old-fashioned husband, a full-time job as a university lab tech, and three demanding children. But her nights
were rarely restful. She suffered from a sleep disorder that was
never precisely diagnosed. She'd wake up screaming, kicking,
thrashing about, sometimes even jumping from her bed, as
though being pursued, landing, with a racing pulse, heavy
breath, in cold sweat, on pillows we placed on the floor for her
protection. My father would try to comfort her, but she was
rarely consolable, largely because she never knew what had happened. We took her to a psychiatrist, who asked my mother if
she was unhappy in her marriage. (My father, speaking for her,
quickly rejected this possibility.) The doctor put her on Valium
and other sedatives that left her groggy and unproductive
and did not help besides, so my mother discontinued them.
Eventually, my parents took to sleeping in separate bedrooms

whenever my father needed to rest. My mother continued to have terror-filled nights for most of her adult life.

I don't remember ever thinking that my mother's dreams could be fatal, but in retrospect, after she got her coronary stent, we should have been more concerned. In a seminal 1923 paper, "Blood Pressure and Heart Action in Sleep and Dreams," John MacWilliam, the Scottish physiologist who identified ventricular fibrillation as the major cause of sudden death, wrote that there are sharp rises in blood pressure, heart rate, and respiration during sleep that exhibit a "suddenness of development." The physiological changes, he wrote, are often more marked than those that occur after running up flights of steps. In his paper, MacWilliam noted that animals experience both sound and disturbed sleep. In the former, blood pressure, heart rate, and respiratory rate decrease as the animals relax into slumber. The latter type of sleep, in contrast, often has violent manifestations: groaning, biting, growling (in dogs), and verbal outbursts. Such changes "imposed sudden and dangerous demands on the heart," and MacWilliam surmised that sudden death could occur, even though the body should be in a state of repose. "In a heart susceptible to fibrillation," he wrote, "a sudden call on the heart during muscular exertion and excitement in the waking state is often fatal. In the disturbed conditions of sleep and dreaming, a similar mechanism is sometimes brought suddenly and strongly into action."

The belief that intense dreams can cause sudden cardiac death is embedded in folklore. In Thailand, for example, "widow ghosts" take men away in the dead of night, according to local legends, and the men have been known to disguise themselves as women at bedtime to protect themselves. However, research into this phenomenon only began about a hundred years ago. We now know that 12 percent of cardiovascular deaths and 14 percent of myocardial infarctions probably occur during sleep, even though victims are ostensibly resting. Intense changes in sympathetic nervous system activity can take place during rapid eye movement, or REM, sleep, when most vivid dreams occur. REM sleep can result in surges of adrenaline that disrupt atherosclerotic plaque, stimulate clotting, and cause coronary spasm and ventricular arrhythmias, which may manifest only after awakening and thus be wrongly attributed to the early-morning period rather than to sleep itself. Especially vulnerable times are 2:00 in the morning, when coronary events seem to peak; 4:00 a.m., when patients with sudden arrhythmias most often die; and the last episode of REM sleep before awakening, which is frequently the most intense of the night. In the latter, breathing often becomes fast and irregular, and blood pressure can rise dramatically. Heart rate may increase from 50 to 170 beats per minute just a few seconds into a nightmare. This is likely what killed my mother.

My mother got her stent in 2006, when she was sixty-four. I often worried she'd be the first in our immediate family to succumb to a heart attack. Heart disease was not her biggest problem, however. In 2011, after several months in which her movements slowed as if she were passing through viscous oil, she was diagnosed with Parkinson's disease. Sinemet, the anti-Parkinson's drug, helped to relieve her muscle rigidity, but her condition quickly declined. She became forgetful. Conversations, once so easy with her, stopped flowing. She stammered, her lips pursing as though she were slurping a thick beverage through a thin straw. Parkinson's also caused dangerous drops in her blood pressure, resulting in frequent falls. After about a year, we pressed our father, who was having his own memory trouble, to retire his genetics professorship in North Dakota and move to Long Island to live closer to me and my brother. When my parents arrived in August 2014, it was alarming how much my mother's situation had deteriorated.

She had become virtually helpless. Nights when I'd visit, my mother would be sitting at the dinner table, papers strewn about, spilling food on her bib. Her precipitous decline no doubt overwhelmed my father, who frequently became enraged, a big change for him. The friend who helped my parents move took me aside after they arrived. "Your father has to have hope," she said.

"Hope for what?" I asked.

"That one day your mother will be able to do the things she can't do right now."

We wanted my mother to remain in her own home, which meant that we—my brother, my sister, and I—were going to have to chip in to help. It was a small price to pay, we thought, for our parents' continuing to live independently. When my sister visited from Minneapolis, she would bathe and dress my mother. I administered her medications and helped with groceries. My brother took care of household issues. Still, my parents' home, like my parents, was in a constant state of disrepair.

Of course, we wanted to do more, but my mother, embarrassed by her disability, felt guilty. One night I was helping her up the steps to her bedroom. She was walking slowly; after several recent spills, she was terrified of falling again. But even as she struggled, her hands turning white as she gripped the banister, she turned to me and said, "This must be so hard for you."

As the workload increased, we hired caregivers—as much for ourselves as for our mother. But after some thefts, we realized we had to be more careful about whom we allowed into our parents' home. One caregiver took an iPhone, silver spoons, and my mother's diamond earrings. I furiously drove to her home in a run-down section of Queens to retrieve the items. She lived in a basement with her two children. The sink was filled with unwashed dishes. Any sudden vibration and tiny roaches would scurry into cracks in the wall. The children watched fearfully as I demanded before an outsized poster of the goddess Lakshmi that the woman return the earrings—my mother was despondent without them—but she steadfastly denied she had taken anything. In the end, I stormed out empty-handed.

My mother's disease progressed. She broke her foot in a fall and spent half a day in the emergency room. She developed staring spells in which she would become unresponsive, causing a new round of panic. More than once we took her to the ER to rule out stroke. Because of Sinemet, she started to have visual hallucinations of insects crawling on her bed or people sleeping on the carpet. She resisted using a bedside commode, so my father was constantly walking her to the bathroom, even in the middle of the night, when we feared she'd fall and break her hip. My mother still had nightmares, but because of the Parkinson's, she could no longer jump out of bed. Eventually, she required a live-in aide to help her with the basic activities of daily living: bathing, feeding, walking, dressing. She once said to me, "Son, do the things you want when you are young. The decline will happen faster than you realize."

We added more and different medications—fludrocortisone for low blood pressure, Seroquel for hallucinations, drugs to treat the side effects of other drugs—with little benefit, never knowing whether our mother would have been better off if we hadn't adjusted the medications in the first place. Even as Parkinson's robbed her of the life she'd enjoyed, a full life raising successful children and managing a household that was always running on overdrive, my mother never asked, why me? But we always said, why her?

After each stepwise decline, she'd insist, "If I can stay like this, it'll be okay." She was able to recalibrate her expectations as her condition deteriorated, leaving her spirit mostly intact. But it was painful to watch. One day my brother, Rajiv, ever the pragmatist, said he wished our mother would die quickly. It was how our maternal grandfather had died, of a myocardial infarction just after his eighty-third birthday, and I remembered my mother had been grateful for the quick and painless demise. But I tore into my brother. I wasn't ready to lose my mother. I wanted her to remain alive for as long as possible.

The morning she died, Rajiv called me from his car. It was an odd hour for him to be calling—I was getting ready to go to work—so I knew something was wrong. "Mom isn't doing well," he said calmly. "I think you should go over there."

I told him I'd go after dropping my kids off at school.

"Go now," he said. "I think Mom just died."

It was a sunny April day. A mild breeze was blowing under a light blue, nearly cloudless sky. Speeding down the road, I called my father. He answered the phone coolly, but when he heard my voice, he started sobbing. He couldn't tell me anything—other than to drive carefully—so I told him to hand the phone to Harwinder, my mother's aide. She told me that she had been awakened at five o'clock in the morning by groans. She called to my mother from her cot across the room, but my mother did not respond. She was about to get up to check on her when my mother took three deep breaths and went silent. She assumed my mother had gone back to sleep—this had happened before during a nightmare—but in the morning when she tried to wake my mother, she did not react. She wasn't breathing; her skin was pale and cold. "She has completed, sir," Harwinder said before I heard my father shout that an ambulance had pulled up outside.

I'd visited my mother the night before. She was having a harder time walking than usual. When I asked, she admitted to feeling mild pressure on the left side of her chest, which I attributed to a recent fall. Now, maddeningly stuck on the road behind a school bus, I realized the chest pain had probably been coronary angina and that my mother had likely died of a heart attack in her sleep. Nothing else could have killed her so quickly.

When I pulled up to my parents' house, there were no cars in the driveway. I ran up to the front door, but it was locked. I frantically rang the doorbell, but no one was home. When I called my brother, he told me the medics had taken my mother to the Plainview Hospital Emergency Room a couple of miles away. He had arrived just in time to prevent them from administering CPR in the back of the ambulance. They had insisted on it—my mother did not have a do-not-resuscitate order—but my brother was adamant, even pulling rank with his hospital ID. He was not going to let them assault our mother. It was plain to see, my brother told them, that she was gone.

In the emergency room, I was led to a curtained-off space where Rajiv, Harwinder, and my father were sitting with my mother. She lay on a gurney, a purple throw draped over her. She had on red nail polish; a bright red bindi still adorned her forehead. My father sat on a stool beside the stretcher, his arms thrown over her body, his head resting on her arm. He touched her hands, massaged her feet. Her mouth was open. He asked me if they would close it for the funeral. "She was so pretty," he said, and then he broke down.

Later that morning, I took Harwinder back to my parents' house so she could prepare it for visitors. As we pulled up, the haze from a neighbor's sprinkler refracted a colorful rainbow, a minor affront on such a solemn day. Inside the house, I managed to make it up to the landing before I was overcome. The fan was still running in my mother's bedroom. Her shawl was hanging on her brass bed frame. The pillow she used to prop up her feet lay under her comforter. Inside the closet was the back massager I'd presented her years before, still in the box; she'd been waiting to open it. On the bedroom floor were the discarded flip tops of drug vials, gauze, and a "smart pad" for checking arrhythmias: the detritus of a futile and aborted resuscitation that the paramedics had left behind. Like both my grandfathers, my mother had succumbed to ventricular fibrillation after a sudden heart attack, though in her case it had happened during sleep. That cardiac death had hit my mother during slumber made the heart seem even more menacing.

In the wet, flat days that followed, there was so much to do—informing friends and relatives, receiving guests, then the funeral and the cremation—there was almost no time to grieve. But once the ceremonies were over, the grief pelted me like waves from the sea, receding periodically only to wash over me once again. At the funeral of a friend's mother two years before, a colleague had said to me, "You never really grow up until your parents die." Now, finally, I understood what he meant. What he meant was, while your parents are alive, there is always someone who thinks of you as a child. When I was a boy, my mother used to tell me a Hindu myth about a man who had been promised the world—unlimited riches—if he would just drown his mother. At the riverbed, as he starts to submerge her in the frigid water, she implores, "Stay out of the water, son! . . . You'll catch a cold." And so it was with my mother. If our family was a body, my mother was its heart: the piece that nourishes and ensures the workings of the rest. On the morning of her funeral, as I was adjusting my tie in front of the mirror, I could almost hear her telling me to stand tall, wear a proper suit, and speak confidently. I remembered the frogs in high school, and I started to cry. I could hear my mother telling me once again, "You should do a different experiment, son. Your heart is too small for this."

In a way, her death was merciful, putting an end to her suffering. But it was sudden, and it left a deep hole. "This world is like that," the proprietor of my mother's favorite sweets shop told me when I visited her. In the prior three months, she had lost her mother-in-law, her brother-in-law, and both her parents. And though I knew many had suffered far worse tragedies than mine, the swiftness of my mother's death gnawed at me. At times, I felt angry: angry that she had been so content to play a supporting role to my father's, resentful of the light touch she had applied to my adult life. And, of course, I felt guilty. She'd complained of chest pains the night before she died. Should I have taken her complaint more seriously? As a cardiologist, I knew that one of every two women will develop heart disease in her lifetime, and one in three will die from it, two-thirds with unrecognized symptoms. Yet in my mother's case, I suffered a blank. Rajiv had no patience with my second-guessing. "I don't want to hear that you made a mistake with Mom," he cried. "You did not, you did not, you did not! We will never know for sure what she died from. All we know is that it was a blessing."

In physiology, there is the concept of referred pain, when an injury to a visceral organ is felt someplace else—as, for example, when heart injury causes arm or jaw pain. And perhaps so it is with emotional pain, too. What I was really feeling was remorse for neglecting my mother in her final days. I had been preoccupied, too focused on my own interests. In her last couple of months, when she was ill and terribly lonely, she would ask me when I was going to come to visit. Then, invariably, she would tell me not to come that day; it was too cold, too hot, or too wet—always something with the weather—and she didn't want me to get sick. After her death, it was a daily struggle trying to keep such regrets from taking hold. But the person who would have fought hardest against them would have been my mother.

I wish she could have seen her funeral, witnessed the scores of friends who came from across the country. For someone who was content to cede the spotlight to her accomplished husband and children, she would have been shocked at how many came to pay their respects, not because of anything she did, but because of who she was, which is perhaps the greatest accomplishment of all.

•

The ashes remained in my father's closet for almost two months. He couldn't decide whether to scatter them in the holy water at Haridwar, on the banks of the Ganges River in India, or in the Atlantic off the shore of Long Island. In the end, he elected not to make the long journey. So Rajiv booked a motorboat in Freeport, and we set off on a bright morning just after Memorial Day to submerge my mother's remains. On a table on the boat, the priest opened a suitcase and arranged the items we would need: incense, cotton balls, the urn, a few edibles. My father, dressed in brown slacks and a yellow shirt, watched quietly. He had never been particularly religious, and it was clear that for him my mother's passing, notwithstanding this last ritual, was over. As the boat sped hard over the waves, my belly churned. I had to keep my waist in contact with the priest's table to keep from falling over.

The priest started off by placing a long piece of red thread on my and my brother's heads, dangling down to our shoulders. He smeared tikkas of red paste on our brows. Next, he lit incense sticks and cotton balls soaked in oil. Rajiv and I made sixteen balls of dough, about the size of a donut hole, from flour, water, and milk and placed them on a metal plate, along with acorns, rice, and an assortment of seeds and other provisions, including holy water from Haridwar, that were supposed to sustain my mother in her journey into the afterlife. The priest unscrewed the top of the urn, and we sprinkled holy water on the plastic bag containing my mother's remains. We then opened the bag and poured in more water and some milk, along with the items on the plate. Next, we emptied the contents of the bag into a white wicker basket. The ashes were charcoal gray; it was hard to believe that this was all that was left of the body. We placed the empty bag in the basket, too. Then we waited for the dust to settle.

The boat slowed to a stop. As the eldest son, Rajiv was given the honor of scattering the ashes, but I wouldn't have been able to do so anyway; by then I was feeling horribly seasick. On the deck, while the priest chanted, his bald pate glistening in the heat, Rajiv placed the wicker basket on a metal hook at the end of a long stick. Then, without ceremony or words—apart from the inscrutable Sanskrit syllables spitting out from the priest's lips— he leaned over the side of the boat and lowered the basket into the water. It had a metal weight to help it sink. I watched it submerge like a head, ghostlike, its contents exploding into a murky cloud in the greenish water. The priest told us to clasp our hands together in prayer. No one said anything as he violently chanted. Then, when he was done, a crew member retrieved the basket with some rope and lifted it back onto the boat. We turned around to head back to shore.

My father rode in the car with me on the way home. We were both tired, and my stomach was just beginning to settle. I put on Beethoven's Piano Sonata no. 8, the *Pathétique*. I looked over at my father. He was staring ahead quietly, listening to the music. He rolled down the window, and a hot wind passed over us. He said nothing for a while; there were only the shrieks and wails of passing cars. Then he said, "We spent our whole life together. I miss her all the time."

14

Compensatory Pause

Satisfaction cannot be stored.
—Peter Sterling, neurobiologist

In 1990, Dean Ornish, a cardiologist at the University of California at San Francisco, and his colleagues published the Lifestyle Heart Trial in the British journal *The Lancet*. In the study, forty-eight patients with moderate-to-severe coronary artery disease were randomly assigned to usual care or an "intensive lifestyle" that included a low-fat vegetarian diet, an hour of daily walking, group psychosocial support, and stress management. After a year, patients in the lifestyle group had a nearly 5 percent reduction in coronary plaque. After five years, the reduction was about 8 percent. Patients who adhered most closely to the program derived the most benefits in an almost dose-dependent relationship. Patients in the group receiving usual care, on the other hand, had an average 5 percent more coronary obstruction after one year and 28 percent after five years. They also had roughly double the rate of cardiac events, including heart attacks, coronary angioplasty, coronary artery bypass surgery, and cardiac-related deaths.

Ornish's study was roundly criticized. It tested a small cohort, reviewers said, hardly representative of the general population. Only half the patients who were invited actually participated, suggesting possible selection bias. Also, virtually none of the patients were on statins or other cholesterol-lowering drugs, so the effect of intensive lifestyle modification on modern, well-treated heart patients was anyone's guess. Moreover, a study published in 2013 in *The New England Journal of Medicine* showed that patients who consume a Mediterranean diet rich in olive oil, fruits and vegetables, fish, and nuts had a roughly 30 percent lower risk of cardiac events, including heart attacks and death, than patients advised to follow a low-fat diet, albeit one less extreme than Ornish's.

Nevertheless, Ornish believed in his results and scaled up his program, eventually offering it at twenty-five hospitals and clinics across the country. He persuaded Medicare to pay for it as a kind of "intensive cardiac rehabilitation." The Ornish plan today consists of two four-hour sessions per week for nine weeks, each comprising an hour-long nutrition class, an hour of exercise, an hour of group support facilitated by a social worker, and an hour of yoga and meditation.

I'd heard Ornish speak about the benefits of his program, so one Friday afternoon in early fall I drove out to the Chambers Center for Well Being in Morristown, New Jersey, the closest Ornish center to where I live, to learn more. I went for a selfish reason. I'd recently learned the results of my CT scan.

When Dr. Trost showed me my coronary blockages, I can't say I was surprised. I'd worried so much about heart disease my whole life that the result seemed almost fated. The disease was still relatively mild, but I knew that most ruptures of coronary plaque—and therefore most heart attacks—occur at places of mild, not severe, narrowing. Mild plaque tends to be softer, thinner, more fat-laden, and possibly more prone to rupture and thrombosis than more advanced plaque.* So I found myself in a clinical catch-22, with a disease too small to fix yet too large

---

*Stress tests cannot tell if a plaque is vulnerable. Even today, no test in medicine can do so reliably.

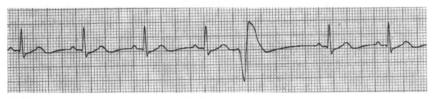

EKG showing a premature ventricular contraction

to ignore. Why had it developed? Was it the few cigarettes I'd smoked in college? Too many pastries and marital spats? Or was the disease programmed into me? Whatever the reason, my future suddenly seemed intolerably unpredictable. I had a peculiar feeling that I wanted to speed up my life to witness the important moments before I ran out of time.

For years, ever since medical school, I've had premature ventricular contractions, a mostly benign condition in which my heart flutters or does a sort of flip-flop when an extra, unexpected beat comes in. Most PVCs are followed by a "compensatory pause," when the next heartbeat is delayed so the heart can get back in step with its normal rhythm. During the compensatory pause, the ventricles fill with blood for a bit longer than usual, so the first beat after a premature one is unusually strong, a thud in the chest to announce the heart's rhythm has gone back to the way it was. As I lay in my den after my scan, listening to the crickets outside, it occurred to me that my scan was like a PVC, an interruption of the normal sequence of things. Was I going to let things go back to the way they were? Or was I going to do a reset?

Over the following days, I underwent more tests. An echocardiogram showed that my heart's chambers and valves were functioning normally. A carotid ultrasound revealed no plaque in the arteries that feed the brain. However, a blood test did show that my level of lipoprotein(a), a cholesterol-carrying molecule, was elevated. A high serum concentration of lipoprotein(a) is associated with more than double the normal risk of developing coronary artery disease or stroke.

Lipoprotein(a) could partially explain the extraordinarily

high rates of heart disease and cardiovascular death among South Asians, but there are other factors. South Asians seem to have smaller coronary arteries than other ethnic groups, which may result in more turbulent blood flow and wall stress that can initiate atherosclerosis. South Asian blood may also contain smaller and denser cholesterol particles that are more prone to causing arterial hardening. The adoption of a "Western" lifestyle—high calories, low exercise—hasn't helped either, possibly activating so-called thrifty genes that create abdominal fat, thus increasing the risk of insulin resistance and diabetes. (These genes might have been advantageous in times of famine, but they are a problem in a world of abundance.) Social and cultural factors undoubtedly play a role, too. This was certainly true of my mother. The culture in which she was brought up discouraged adults from taking time for themselves, away from the responsibilities of job, home, and children, to exercise. Moreover, like many of her Indian friends, my mother believed in fate, that her future—and future health—were preordained. Saddled by this fatalistic philosophy, she never believed that one could change the natural course of one's life.

But I did not want my CT scan to be my fate. I wanted to make changes to try to stabilize—or possibly even reverse—the damage. But what sorts of changes were needed? I was already leading a pretty healthy life. I was taking a cholesterol-lowering statin prophylactically. The changes, I realized, were going to have to be more fundamental.

I called my friend Anand, a television producer and a yogi, who suggested getting together one evening after work at the Hindu temple in Flushing. It was a warm midsummer evening when we met. The temple is in a middle-class neighborhood of single-family homes partitioned by rusty chain-link fences. A sign out front reminded patrons, "Do not break coconut here." When I arrived, a prayer ceremony was just ending. A man clad in a white dhoti was clanging a bell and fervently chanting, "Shanti, shanti, shanti . . ." I spotted Anand, a paunchy, middle-aged fellow, wearing beige kurta pajamas and with a streak of

red powder on his forehead. Head bowed, he moved purposefully from one garlanded statue to the next, kneeling at each to
murmur a few words. When he was finished, he came over and
shook my hand. Then we went downstairs to the canteen, where
we ordered *dosas* and sweet *lassi* and sat down at a cafeteria-
style table to wait for our food.

I felt as if I should explain why I had called him, but Anand
seemed to require no explanation. He sat contentedly, taking
in the busy room. After some polite chitchat, I told him about
my scan. Brow furrowed, he listened carefully in the manner of
a psychoanalyst.

"I have always found you take things very seriously," Anand
finally said. In his mind, my scan results no doubt were related
to this. "Learn to get out of your mind."

I laughed. "And how does one do that?"

His face turned serious. "Yoga, meditation, a walk in the
park, whatever works. When you are doing it, you think it is a
waste of time, but it is the most valuable time because it is helping you manage the whole day."

I'd tried yoga a few times. After Sonia and I were married,
we'd ventured down to a drab studio in Tribeca, where a *mala*-
necklaced old woman made us stand in painful poses while we
focused on a spot on a pitted wall. I did feel more relaxed afterward (probably acute respiratory alkalosis brought on by deep
breathing, I'd hypothesized), but I hadn't kept up with the
practice.

Anand advised returning to it. "Look at this scan as a blessing," he said encouragingly. "It will help you find ways to become more composed. Your mind, your thoughts, are not your
owner, but they are behaving as your owner. Go beyond mind.
That is the only place you are truly free."

•

And so I found myself in Morristown, New Jersey. The Ornish
facility was in a large office complex just off a densely wooded
road. The giant oak trees were already dropping their leaves into

colorful piles. Carole, the nurse practitioner who runs the program, met me at the front desk when I arrived. "We've had quite a few young Indian men call us," she'd told me when we spoke on the phone.

The sessions were over for the day, so Carole gave me a tour of the facility: the kitchen, with its polished stovetops, where participants spend an hour together having a vegetarian lunch; the gym, supervised by two nurse practitioners and an exercise physiologist, where a few stalwarts were still running on treadmills; and the stress management room, where chairs were arranged in a circle and yoga mats were still on the floor. Carole told me her father was seventy when he was diagnosed with heart disease. He'd been having pains in his shoulder, and though a stress test was normal, a coronary angiogram revealed triple-vessel disease that was so advanced, surgery or angioplasty was no longer an option. "He was living on threads," she said. With no treatment alternatives, her father tried the Ornish program. He followed it for two months before dying suddenly of an arrhythmia. Despite this morbid introduction, Carole had been working in Ornish-style preventive cardiology ever since.

In her office, Carole showed me angiograms of program participants whose coronary disease had regressed. "When people talk about the Ornish program, they usually talk about the diet," she said. "But the social support and stress management are probably the most important pieces." Patients were often reluctant to participate in group therapy, she said. "Some ask for a waiver. They don't want to open up to strangers. But it almost always ends up being their favorite part."

Ornish himself puts a great premium on the psychosocial piece of his program. He has pointed out, for example, that some patients in his original control group adopted diet and exercise plans that were almost as intense as those of the intervention group. However, their heart disease still progressed; diet and exercise alone weren't enough to facilitate coronary plaque regression. At both one- and five-year follow-ups, stress management was more strongly correlated with reversal of coronary artery disease than exercise. "The need for connection and community often goes unfulfilled in our culture," Ornish said in a 2015 interview. "We know that these things affect the quality of our lives, but they also affect our survival to a much larger degree than most people realize."

Many studies have suggested that Ornish is probably right. In one example, patients who were depressed after a heart attack were four times as likely to die within six months as those who were not, irrespective of usual Framingham risk factors like high cholesterol, hypertension, obesity, and smoking. In another study, menopausal women with no history of cardiovascular disease who expressed more hopelessness on a psychological questionnaire had more carotid artery thickening and an older vascular age than matched patients who felt good about their lives.* No doubt many of these studies are small, and of course correlation does not prove causation; it is certainly possible that stress leads to unhealthy habits—poor nutrition, less physical activity, more smoking—and this is the real reason for the increased cardiovascular risk. But as with the association of smoking with lung cancer, when so many studies show the same thing and there are mechanisms to explain a causal relationship, it seems perverse to deny that one probably exists. What Ornish and others have concluded is fully consistent with what I have learned in my two decades in medicine: that the emotional heart affects its biological counterpart in multiple mysterious ways.

Carole told me she uses "trackers" to see how well patients follow the program on the days they do not come to the center. There are trackers for diet and exercise, of course, but also ones for love and support. Patients are asked to rate "How connected am I?" on a simple numerical scale. Those who do more

---

*Women measuring higher on the hopelessness scale had more carotid thickening, equal to the amount caused by one year of aging.

than one hour of stress management daily have the greatest improvement in coronary blood flow. "We run our lives at such a frenetic pace," Carole said. "Our sympathetic nervous systems are on overdrive. But how we react to the stress is under our control."

Unfortunately, I was not going to be able to participate in the Ornish program. Traveling to New Jersey twice a week for nearly three months wasn't feasible, and abridged courses, Carole sadly informed me, were not yet available. She promised to send me some material so I could get started on my own. "Try to find joy in each day," she said, walking me to the elevator. "Instead of thinking about the past or worrying about the future, focus on the present." I told her I would do my best. Then I went down to the parking lot, got into my car, and joined the Friday evening rush toward Long Island.

•

Perhaps more than any other area of medicine, cardiology has been at the forefront of technological innovation and quality improvement over the past fifty years. This golden period has witnessed a barrage of life-prolonging advances, many of them discussed in this book, including implantable pacemakers and defibrillators, coronary angioplasty, coronary bypass surgery, and heart transplantation. Preventive health initiatives, such as smoking cessation and cholesterol and blood pressure reduction, have supplemented these biomedical advances. The result has been a 60 percent drop in cardiovascular mortality since 1968, the year I was born. There are few stories in twentieth-century medicine that have been as uplifting or far-reaching.

For a while it appeared that cancer would replace heart disease as the leading cause of death in the United States, but no more. The rate of decline in cardiovascular mortality has slowed significantly in the past decade. There are many reasons for this. The fall in smoking rates has leveled off. Americans have become more overweight. Diabetes cases are projected to nearly double in the next twenty-five years. But I believe there is another reason, too. Cardiology in its current form might have reached the limits of what it can do to prolong life.

This would have been heresy to pioneers like Walt Lillehei, Andreas Gruentzig, and Michel Mirowski, but today it is hard to refute. The law of diminishing returns applies to every human enterprise, and cardiovascular medicine is no different. For instance, ever since coronary thrombosis was shown to be the cause of most heart attacks, cardiologists have taken it as an article of faith that more rapid treatment of such thromboses improves patient survival. "Time is muscle," goes the operative mantra, and the shorter the delay, the better. Yet a study of nearly 100,000 patients published in 2013 in *The New England Journal of Medicine* found that shorter "door-to-balloon" times—the period from a patient's hospital presentation to inflation of a balloon to restore coronary blood flow—did not improve in-hospital survival. The median door-to-balloon time dropped to sixty-seven minutes, from eighty-three, in the period studied, but short-term death rates did not change.

There are several plausible explanations for this result. Perhaps heart attack patients who are healthier and at low risk for death are already getting expeditious treatment, and those who are at higher risk are experiencing the most delays. Perhaps the follow-up time in the study was too short, and if we waited a bit longer, a survival benefit would be seen. Or perhaps there is another reason. Mortality after a heart attack has already dropped tenfold, from 30 percent to 3 percent, since Mason Sones invented coronary angiography in 1958. Can the tweaking or speeding up of existing procedures possibly yield any significant additional benefit?

There are other examples of such diminishing returns. In my specialty, heart failure, medications such as beta-blockers and ACE inhibitors have profoundly improved survival since their advent in the mid-1980s. Yet recent studies of newer agents—endothelin blockers, vasopressin antagonists—have shown little benefit. Today patients' Framingham risk factors, such as hypertension and high cholesterol, are better controlled. It is getting harder to improve on existing successes.

No doubt we should celebrate the rise of high-tech medicine. For example, more than 90 percent of patients who present directly to hospitals that do angioplasty have door-to-balloon times today of less than ninety minutes, with a median time of approximately sixty minutes, a major improvement from only a few years ago. However, this means that the bar is continually being set higher for every new treatment.

I believe that cardiovascular medicine in its current form, focusing on investigating minor iterations of commonly used drugs or add-on therapies or optimizing existing procedures, will increasingly produce only marginal advances in the years ahead. We will need to shift to a new paradigm, one focused on prevention—turning down the faucet rather than mopping up the floor—to continue to make the kind of progress to which patients and doctors have become accustomed. In this paradigm, psychosocial factors will need to be front and center in how we think about health problems. Despite the centuries-old association of the heart with emotions, this is still a domain that remains largely unexplored. However, today it is increasingly clear that chronic diseases like hypertension, diabetes, and heart failure are inextricably linked to the state of our neighborhoods, jobs, families, and minds.

Heart disease, as we've seen, has psychological, social, and even political roots. To treat our hearts optimally will require interventions on all these fronts. This is much easier said than done, of course. Psychosocial "repair" is just as prone to unexpected consequences, difficult trade-offs, conflicting values, and diminishing returns as any medical treatment. We cannot even agree on what should be repaired. But we will have to find ways, as Peter Sterling, the neurobiologist, has put it, to "reduce the need for vigilance and to restore small satisfactions," such as our contact with nature and with one another. For some, this will require city-planning initiatives to encourage walking or bicycling, for example, instead of more sedentary lifestyles. Others will require fortification in more social realms, such as the enhancement of public life. For still others, cardiovascular benefits will come from more individualistic pursuits, such as yoga and meditation. Whatever the case, it is increasingly clear today that the biological heart is inextricably linked to its metaphorical counterpart. To treat our hearts, we must repair our societies and minds. We must look at not only our bodies but also ourselves.

•

I am lying on a blanket, staring up at the stars. Though the sun set more than an hour ago, the sky is fringed with streaks of orange. The air is still and smells of citronella and bug spray. Though the party is winding down, children continue to play in a sugar-fueled frenzy, barreling down inflatable slides and running tag on the lawn. My daughter, Pia, is sitting on my chest, burrowing her head affectionately into my neck. "Are you happy?" she asks me, her warm breath tickling my skin.

"Yes," I reply. "Are you?"

"Yes, Dad," she says. "I'm happy, too."

As another summer winds down, my CT scan is a distant memory. It was supposed to change everything, but in the end it was a hiccup, a PVC, and my life has returned to its normal rhythm. Like when you plan a trip somewhere and you think the place will feel different, the way you see it in pictures, and then you get there and it's the same as the place you came from: same sky, same air, same clouds. Of course, I've made changes. I exercise almost every day now, and I eat better, too. I spend more time with my children and with friends. I still enjoy working hard, but I am no longer so contemptuous of relaxation.

Many factors that affect our health are out of our direct control—we cannot diminish the stress that comes with reading the newspaper, or with supporting a family in a competitive economy, or with living in a violent neighborhood—at least not without patient and collective effort. But many entail decisions, and ways of behaving, that we can master. Do you want to live a long, healthy, and prosperous life? Don't smoke. Exercise. Eat right. But also take good care of your interpersonal relationships and the way you deal with life's inevitable upsets and traumas. Your mind-set, your coping strategies, how you navigate challenging circumstances, your capacity to transcend distress, your capacity to love—these things, I believe, are also a matter of life and death.

I imagine I'll repeat the CT scan at some point to see whether my coronary plaque has progressed. But I am not all that afraid of what I will find. I feel reassured by the knowledge that has accumulated in my field over the past century, even the past decade. We can now replace heart valves without open-heart surgery. We can inject stem cells to heal damaged heart muscle. My paternal grandfather was in his early fifties when he died. I am forty-eight as I write these words. But I am not my grandfather. I am privileged to live in an era in which the human heart has yielded to the human hand. The three-centimeter trip took millennia, starting ostensibly from the pericardium but really from a time when the heart was an almost supernatural object surrounded by taboos. Through this journey, the heart was transformed into a machine that can be manipulated and controlled. But these manipulations, as we have learned, must be complemented by attention to the emotional life that the heart, for thousands of years, was believed to contain.

After so many years in the business, I see heart shapes everywhere: in the splash of raindrops on my windshield, in the beets I slice in my kitchen, in strawberry slivers and bitten cherries. And every morning, the drops of milk at the swirling center of my coffee cup make a spiral wave.

I still often think of my grandfathers and of course my mother. I can picture my paternal grandfather slumping in cardiac arrest onto that stone floor in Kanpur, surrounded by his alarmed family. Or my maternal grandfather sitting in his drawing room in New Delhi on the day he died, listening to the news on the BBC while waiting for his breakfast. In the span of a few heartbeats, he was no more. Though the mechanisms of their deaths (and probably my mother's) were the same, the outcomes were so different. One death left enduring trauma, the other two gratitude for a merciful demise. For much of my life, I feared the heart's power, but I don't see it as I once did. Yes, the heart can snuff out your life, but when the pressure of existence builds up, this organ, prime mover and citadel, is also a safety valve that can facilitate a quick and humane end.

Supplementary Reading

INTRODUCTION: THE ENGINE OF LIFE
Ford, Earl S., Umed A. Ajani, Janet B. Croft, Julia A. Critchley, Darwin R.
    Labarthe, Thomas E. Kottke, Wayne H. Giles, and Simon Capewell.
    "Explaining the Decrease in U.S. Deaths from Coronary Disease,
    1980–2000." *The New England Journal of Medicine* 356, no. 23 (2007):
    2388–98.

1. A SMALL HEART
Cannon, Walter B. "'Voodoo' Death." *American Anthropologist* 44, no. 2
    (1942): 169–81.
Hall, Joan Lord. "'To the Very Heart of Loss': Rival Constructs of 'Heart' in
    Antony and Cleopatra." *College Literature* 18, no. 1 (1991): 64–76.
Kriegbaum, Margit, Ulla Christensen, Per Kragh Andersen, Merete Osler, and
    Rikke Lund. "Does the Association Between Broken Partnership and
    First Time Myocardial Infarction Vary with Time After Break-Up?"
    International Journal of Epidemiology 42, no. 6 (2013): 1811–19.
Leor, Jonathan, W. Kenneth Poole, and Robert A. Kloner. "Sudden Cardiac
    Death Triggered by an Earthquake." *The New England Journal of Med-
    icine* 334, no. 7 (1996): 413–19.
McCraty, Rollin. "Heart-Brain Neurodynamics: The Making of Emotions."
    HeartMath Research Center, HeartMath Institute. Publication 03-015
    (2003).
Nager, Frank. *The Mythology of the Heart.* Basel: Roche, 1993.
Richter, Curt P. "On the Phenomenon of Sudden Death in Animal and Man."
    Psychosomatic Medicine 19, no. 3 (1957): 191–98.

Rosch, Paul J. "Why the Heart Is Much More Than a Pump." HeartMath Library Archives.

Samuels, Martin A. "The Brain–Heart Connection." *Circulation* 116 (2007): 77–84.

Weiss, M. "Signifying the Pandemics: Metaphors of AIDS, Cancer, and Heart Disease." *Medical Anthropology Quarterly*, n.s., no. 11 (1997): 456–76.

Yawger, N. S. "Emotions as the Cause of Rapid and Sudden Death." *Archives of Neurology and Psychiatry* 36 (1936): 875–79.

2. PRIME MOVER

Harvey, William. "On the Motion of the Heart and Blood in Animals." Translated by R. Willis. In *Scientific Papers: Physiology, Medicine, Surgery, Geology, with Introductions, Notes, and Illustrations*. New York: P. F. Collier and Son, 1910.

O'Malley, C. D. *Andreas Vesalius of Brussels, 1514–1564*. Berkeley: University of California Press, 1964.

Park, K. "The Criminal and the Saintly Body: Autopsy and Dissection in Renaissance Italy." *Renaissance Quarterly* 47 (1994): 1–33.

Pasipoularides, A. "Galen, Father of Systematic Medicine: An Essay on the Evolution of Modern Medicine and Cardiology." *International Journal of Cardiology* 172 (2014): 47–58.

Rosch, Paul J. "Why the Heart Is Much More Than a Pump." HeartMath Library Archives.

Schultz, Stanley G. "William Harvey and the Circulation of the Blood: The Birth of a Scientific Revolution and Modern Physiology." *Physiology* 17, no. 5 (2002): 175–80.

Shoja, Mohammadali M., Paul S. Agutter, Marios Loukas, Brion Benninger, Ghaffar Shokouhi, Husain Namdar, Kamyar Ghabili, Majid Khalili, and R. Shane Tubbs. "Leonardo da Vinci's Studies of the Heart." *International Journal of Cardiology* 167, no. 4 (2013): 1126–33.

West, John B. "Marcello Malpighi and the Discovery of the Pulmonary Capillaries and Alveoli." *American Journal of Physiology—Lung, Cellular, and Molecular Physiology* 304, no. 6 (2013): L383–L390.

3. CLUTCH

Alexi-Meskishvili, V., and W. Bottcher. "Suturing of Penetrating Wounds to the Heart in the Nineteenth Century: The Beginnings of Heart Surgery." *The Annals of Thoracic Surgery* 92, no. 5 (2011): 1926–31.

Asensio, Juan A., B. Montgomery Stewart, James Murray, Arthur H. Fox, Andres Falabella, Hugo Gomez, Adrian Ortega, Clark B. Fuller, and

Morris D. Kerstein. "Penetrating Cardiac Injuries." *Surgical Clinics of North America* 76, no. 4 (1996): 685–724.

Cobb, W. Montague. "Daniel Hale Williams—Pioneer and Innovator." *Journal of the National Medical Association* 36, no. 5 (1944): 158.

Dunn, Rob. *The Man Who Touched His Own Heart.* New York: Little, Brown, 2015.

Johnson, Stephen L. *The History of Cardiac Surgery, 1896–1955.* Baltimore: Johns Hopkins University Press, 1970.

Meriwether, Louise. *The Heart Man: Dr. Daniel Hale Williams.* Englewood Cliffs, N.J.: Prentice-Hall, 1972.

Werner, Orla J., Christian Sohns, Aron F. Popov, Jannik Haskamp, and Jan D. Schmitto. "Ludwig Rehn (1849–1930): The German Surgeon Who Performed the Worldwide First Successful Cardiac Operation." *Journal of Medical Biography* 20, no. 1 (2012): 32–34.

4. DYNAMO

Goor, Daniel A. *The Genius of C. Walton Lillehei and the True History of Open Heart Surgery.* New York: Vantage Press, 2007.

Lillehei, C. W. "The Birth of Open Heart Surgery: Then the Golden Years." *Cardiovascular Surgery* 2, no. 3 (1994): 308–17.

Lillehei, C. W., M. Cohen, H. E. Warden, N. R. Ziegler, and R. L. Varco. "The Results of Direct Vision Closure of Ventricular Septal Defects in Eight Patients by Means of Controlled Cross-circulation." *Surgery, Gynecology, and Obstetrics* 101 (1955): 446.

Miller, G. Wayne. *King of Hearts: The True Story of the Maverick Who Pioneered Open Heart Surgery.* New York: Crown, 2000.

Rosenberg, J. C., and C. W. Lillehei. "The Emergence of Cardiac Surgery." *Lancet* 80 (1960): 201–14.

5. PUMP

Brock, R. C. "The Surgery of Pulmonary Stenosis," *British Medical Journal,* no. 2 (1949): 399–406.

Castillo, Javier G., and George Silvay. "John H. Gibbon Jr. and the 60th Anniversary of the First Successful Heart-Lung Machine." *Journal of Cardiothoracic and Vascular Anesthesia* 27, no. 2 (2013): 203–207.

Cohn, Lawrence H. "Fifty Years of Open-Heart Surgery." *Circulation* 1007 (2003): 2168–70.

Gibbon, John H., Jr. "Development of the Artificial Heart and Lung Extracorporeal Blood Circuit." *JAMA* 206, no. 9 (1968): 1983–86.

———. "The Early Development of an Extracorporeal Circulation with an Artificial Heart and Lung." *Transactions of the American Society for Artificial Internal Organs* 13, no. 1 (1967): 77–79.

———. "The Gestation and Birth of an Idea." *Philadelphia Medicine* 13 (1963): 913–16.

Shumacker, Harris B., Jr. *The Evolution of Cardiac Surgery.* Bloomington: Indiana University Press, 1992.

———. *John Heysham Gibbon, Jr., 1903–1973: A Biographical Memoir.* Washington, D.C.: National Academy of Sciences, 1982.

Stoney, William S. "Evolution of Cardiopulmonary Bypass." *Circulation* 119, no. 21 (2009): 2844–53.

6. NUT

Altman, Lawrence K. *Who Goes First? The Story of Self-Experimentation in Medicine.* New York: Random House, 1987.

Forssmann, Werner. *Experiments on Myself.* New York: St. Martin's Press, 1974.

Forssmann-Falck, Renate. "Werner Forssmann: A Pioneer of Cardiology." *American Journal of Cardiology* 79, no. 5 (1997): 651–60.

7. STRESS FRACTURES

Friedman, Meyer, and Ray H. Rosenman. *Type A Behavior and Your Heart.* New York: Alfred A. Knopf, 1974.

Kannel, William B. "Contribution of the Framingham Study to Preventive Cardiology." *Journal of the American College of Cardiology* 15, no. 1 (1990): 206–11.

Kannel, William B., Thomas R. Dawber, Abraham Kagan, Nicholas Revotskie, and Joseph Stokes. "Factors of Risk in the Development of Coronary Heart Disease—Six-Year Follow-Up Experience: The Framingham Study." *Annals of Internal Medicine* 55, no. 1 (1961): 33–50.

Kannel, William B., Tavia Gordon, and Melvin J. Schwartz. "Systolic Versus Diastolic Blood Pressure and Risk of Coronary Heart Disease: The Framingham Study." *American Journal of Cardiology* 27, no. 4 (1971): 335–46.

Kaplan, J. R., S. B. Manuck, T. B. Clarkson, F. M. Lusso, D. M. Taub, and E. W. Miller. "Social Stress and Atherosclerosis in Normocholesterolemic Monkeys." *Science* 220, no. 4598 (1983): 733–35.

Kriegbaum, Margit, Ulla Christensen, Per Kragh Andersen, Merete Osler, and Rikke Lund. "Does the Association Between Broken Partnership and First Time Myocardial Infarction Vary with Time After Break-Up?" *International Journal of Epidemiology* 42, no. 6 (2013): 1811–19.

Mahmood, Syed S., Daniel Levy, Ramachandran S. Vasan, and Thomas J. Wang. "The Framingham Heart Study and the Epidemiology of Cardiovascular Disease: A Historical Perspective." *Lancet* 383, no. 9921 (2014): 999–1008.

Marmot, Michael G. "Health in an Unequal World." *Lancet* 368, no. 9952 (2006): 2081–94.

Marmot, Michael G., and S. Leonard Syme. "Acculturation and Coronary Heart Disease in Japanese-Americans." *American Journal of Epidemiology* 104, no. 3 (1976): 225–47.

Nerem, Robert M., Murina J. Levesque, and J. Fredrick Cornhill. "Social Environment as a Factor in Diet-Induced Atherosclerosis." *Science* 208, no. 4451 (1980): 1475–76.

Oldfield, Benjamin J., and David S. Jones. "Languages of the Heart: The Biomedical and the Metaphorical in American Fiction." *Perspectives in Biology and Medicine* 57, no. 3 (2014): 424–42.

Oppenheimer, Gerald M. "Becoming the Framingham Study, 1947–1950." *American Journal of Public Health* 95, no. 4 (2005): 602–10.

Ramsay, Michael A. E. "John Snow, MD: Anaesthetist to the Queen of England and Pioneer Epidemiologist." *Baylor University Medical Center Proceedings* 19, no. 1 (2006): 24.

Sterling, Peter. "Principles of Allostasis: Optimal Design, Predictive Regulation, Pathophysiology, and Rational Therapeutics." In *Allostasis, Homeostasis, and the Costs of Physiological Adaptation*, edited by Jay Schulkin. New York: Cambridge University Press, 2004.

Worth, Robert M., Hiroo Kato, George G. Rhoads, Abraham Kagan, and Sherman Leonard Syme. "Epidemiologic Studies of Coronary Heart Disease and Stroke in Japanese Men Living in Japan, Hawaii, and California: Mortality." *American Journal of Epidemiology* 102, no. 6 (1975): 481–90.

8. PIPES

Monagan, David, and David O. Williams. *Journey into the Heart: A Tale of Pioneering Doctors and Their Race to Transform Cardiovascular Medicine.* New York: Gotham, 2007.

Mueller, Richard L., and Timothy A. Sanborn. "The History of Interventional Cardiology: Cardiac Catheterization, Angioplasty, and Related Interventions." *American Heart Journal* 129, no. 1 (1995): 146–72.

Payne, Misty M. "Charles Theodore Dotter: The Father of Invention." *Texas Heart Institute* 28, no. 1 (2001): 28.

Rösch, Josef, Frederick S. Keller, and John A. Kaufman. "The Birth, Early

Years, and Future of Interventional Radiology." *Journal of Vascular and Interventional Radiology* 14, no. 7 (2003): 841–53.

Sheldon, William C. "F. Mason Sones, Jr.—Stormy Petrel of Cardiology." *Clinical Cardiology* 17, no. 7 (1994): 405–407.

9. WIRES

Davidenko, Jorge M., Arcady V. Pertsov, Remy Salomonsz, William Baxter, and José Jalife. "Stationary and Drifting Spiral Waves of Excitation in Isolated Cardiac Muscle." *Nature* 355, no. 6358 (1992): 349–51.

De Silva, Regis A. "George Ralph Mines, Ventricular Fibrillation, and the Discovery of the Vulnerable Period." *Journal of the American College of Cardiology* 29, no. 6 (1997): 1397–402.

Garfinkel, Alan, Peng-Sheng Chen, Donald O. Walter, Hrayr S. Karagueuzian, Boris Kogan, Steven J. Evans, Mikhail Karpoukhin, Chun Hwang, Takumi Uchida, Masamichi Gotoh, Obi Nwasokwa, Philip Sager, and James N. Weiss. "Quasiperiodicity and Chaos in Cardiac Fibrillation." *Journal of Clinical Investigation* 99, no. 2 (1997): 305–14.

Garfinkel, Alan, Young-Hoon Kim, Olga Voroshilovsky, Zhilin Qu, Jong R. Kil, Moon-Hyoung Lee, Hrayr S. Karagueuzian, James N. Weiss, and Peng-Sheng Chen. "Preventing Ventricular Fibrillation by Flattening Cardiac Restitution." *Proceedings of the National Academy of Sciences* 97, no. 11 (2000): 6061–66.

Gray, Richard A., José Jalife, Alexandre Panfilov, William T. Baxter, Cándido Cabo, Jorge M. Davidenko, and Arkady M. Pertsov. "Nonstationary Vortex-Like Reentrant Activity as a Mechanism of Polymorphic Ventricular Tachycardia in the Isolated Rabbit Heart." *Circulation* 91, no. 9 (1995): 2454–69.

Link, Mark S., et al. "An Experimental Model of Sudden Death Due to Low-Energy Chest-Wall Impact (Commotio Cordis)." *The New England Journal of Medicine* 338, no. 25 (1998): 1805–11.

MacWilliam, John A. "Cardiac Failure and Sudden Death." *British Medical Journal* 1, no. 1462 (1889): 6.

Mines, George Ralph. "On Circulating Excitations in Heart Muscles and Their Possible Relation to Tachycardia and Fibrillation." *Transactions of the Royal Society of Canada* 8 (1914): 43–52.

Myerburg, Robert J., Kenneth M. Kessler, and Agustin Castellanos. "Pathophysiology of Sudden Cardiac Death." *Pacing and Clinical Electrophysiology* 14, no. 5 (1991): 935–43.

Ruelle, David, and Floris Takens. "On the Nature of Turbulence." *Communications in Mathematical Physics* 20, no. 3 (1971): 167–92.

Winfree, Arthur T. "Electrical Turbulence in Three-Dimensional Heart Muscle." *Science* 206 (1994): 1003–1006.

———. "Sudden Cardiac Death: A Problem in Topology?" *Scientific American* 248, no. 5 (1983): 144–61.

10. GENERATOR

Heilman, M. S. "Collaboration with Michel Mirowski on the Development of the AICD." *Pacing and Clinical Electrophysiology* 14, no. 5 (1991): 910–15.

Jeffrey, Kirk. *Machines in Our Hearts: The Cardiac Pacemaker, the Implantable Defibrillator, and American Health Care.* Baltimore: Johns Hopkins University Press, 2001.

Kinney, Martha Pat. "Knickerbocker, G. Guy." Science Heroes. www.scienceheroes.com/index.php?option=com_content&view=article&id=338&Itemid=284.

Mirowski, M., et al. "Termination of Malignant Ventricular Arrhythmias with an Implanted Automatic Defibrillator in Human Beings." *The New England Journal of Medicine* 303, no. 6 (1980): 322–24.

Mower, Morton M. "Building the AICD with Michel Mirowski." *Pacing and Clinical Electrophysiology* 14, no. 5 (1991): 928–34.

Worthington, Janet Farrar. "The Engineer Who Could." *Hopkins Medical News* (Winter 1998).

11. REPLACEMENT PARTS

Cooley, Denton A. "The Total Artificial Heart as a Bridge to Cardiac Transplantation: Personal Recollections." *Texas Heart Institute Journal* 28, no. 3 (2001): 200.

DeVries, William C., Jeffrey L. Anderson, Lyle D. Joyce, Fred L. Anderson, Elizabeth H. Hammond, Robert K. Jarvik, and Willem J. Kolff. "Clinical Use of the Total Artificial Heart." *The New England Journal of Medicine* 310, no. 5 (1984): 273–78.

McCrae, Donald. *Every Second Counts: The Race to Transplant the First Human Heart.* New York: G. P. Putnam's Sons, 2006.

"Norman Shumway, Heart Transplantation Pioneer, Dies at 83." Stanford Medicine News Center, Feb. 10, 2007. med.stanford.edu/news/all-news/2006/02/norman-shumway-heart-transplantation-pioneer-dies-at-83.html.

Perciaccante, A., M. A. Riva, A. Coralli, P. Charlier, and R. Bianucci. "The Death of Balzac (1799–1850) and the Treatment of Heart Failure During the Nineteenth Century." *Journal of Cardiac Failure* 22, no. 11 (2016): 930–33.

Strauss, Michael J. "The Political History of the Artificial Heart." *The New England Journal of Medicine* 310, no. 5 (1984): 332–36.

Woolley, F. Ross. "Ethical Issues in the Implantation of the Artificial Heart." *The New England Journal of Medicine* 310, no. 5 (1984): 292–96.

12. VULNERABLE HEART

Lown, Bernard. *The Lost Art of Healing.* Boston: Houghton Mifflin, 1996.

Sears, Samuel F., Jamie B. Conti, Anne B. Curtis, Tara L. Saia, Rebecca Foote, and Francis Wen. "Affective Distress and Implantable Cardioverter Defibrillators: Cases for Psychological and Behavioral Interventions." *Pacing and Clinical Electrophysiology* 2, no. 12 (1999): 1831–34.

13. A MOTHER'S HEART

De Silva, Regis A. "John MacWilliam, Evolutionary Biology, and Sudden Cardiac Death." *Journal of the American College of Cardiology* 14, no. 7 (1989): 1843–49.

14. COMPENSATORY PAUSE

Dimsdale, Joel E. "Psychological Stress and Cardiovascular Disease." *Journal of the American College of Cardiology* 51, no. 13 (2008): 1237–46.

Acknowledgments

I am deeply indebted to so many for their help and support in the writing of this book, but none more so than the patients I've had the privilege to care for and learn from during my years as a physician.

My agent, Todd Shuster, has been a friend and an ally for almost two decades. He made me believe that I could write books.

I owe a debt of gratitude to my brilliant editor, Alex Star, who had a clear vision for this book when we first discussed it over lunch. "It will be about the heart, not the heart doctor," he continually reminded me. "We will get closer to our own hearts by reading this book." Alex's editorial acumen is present throughout. I was very lucky to work with him.

I also wish to thank several other colleagues at Farrar, Straus and Giroux: Dominique Lear, who attended to so many important details during the publication process; Jonathan Lippincott, who managed the design; Nick Courage, who created my website; Ingrid Sterner, my copy editor; Susan Goldfarb, my production editor; Scott Borchert; Laury Frieber; and my wonderful publicity team: Jeff Seroy, Brian Gittis, Sarita Varma, and Daniel del Valle.

And of course I am indebted to Jonathan Galassi and Eric Chinski for giving me the chance to write the book in the first place.

I have had the enormous privilege of writing for *The New York Times* for two decades. I am grateful to the many editors there who have helped shape me as a writer, but I owe a special thanks to the preternaturally smart Jamie Ryerson, my op-ed page editor, who has pushed me in my journalism as much as anyone I've worked with.

I am lucky to have a tremendous group of colleagues where I work. I especially want to thank Tamara Jansz, my dear friend; Kim Hammond; Maureen Hogan; Tracey Spruill; and Mickey Katz. I am also grateful to Barry Kaplan, Michael Dowling, David Battinelli, and Lawrence Smith for their ongoing support of my writing.

Several other friends and assistants have earned my heartfelt appreciation, including Eugenie L-Shiah, Angela Goddard, Elias Altman, Sarah Tanchuck, Abbey Wolf, Lisa DeBenedettis, Sung Lee, and Paul Elie. They all critiqued early drafts of the manuscript or assisted me with research. Two assistants stand out for special recognition, Cody Elkhechen and Isabella Gomes, for their intense devotion to the manuscript and for making countless helpful suggestions.

Of course, I am ultimately responsible for these contents. If there are any mistakes, the fault is mine and mine alone.

I save my deepest gratitude for my family: my father, Prem, and my dear sister, Suneeta; my mother, Raj, whom I will always miss; and my brother, Rajiv, who was a deep reservoir of support throughout the entire enterprise. I am also grateful to my wife Sonia's family for their love and support.

Before I had kids, my mother told me, "You can never understand just how much you will love them." She was right. My son, Mohan, is my right-hand man. My darling Pia was the first to tell me to write a book about the heart. They are the twin lights of my life.

Finally, I am ever grateful to my dear wife, Sonia, my partner for twenty years, my love, my toughest critic, and the one person without whom my life would not be.

Index

A NOTE ABOUT THE AUTHOR

Sandeep Jauhar, MD, PhD, is the director of the Heart Failure Program at Long Island Jewish Medical Center. He is the bestselling author of *Doctored* and *Intern* and a *New York Times* contributing op-ed writer. He lives with his wife and their son and daughter on Long Island.

31901064538160